Vegetarian Pregnancy

Also by Sharon K. Yntema

Vegetarian Baby
Vegetarian Children

Vegetarian Pregnancy

*The definitive nutritional guide
to having a healthy baby*

Sharon K. Yntema

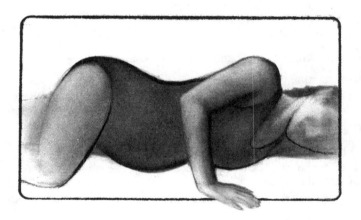

Illustrated by William M. Benson

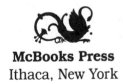

McBooks Press
Ithaca, New York

The author and the publisher believe that this book outlines an excellent regimen for a healthy pregnancy. However, they cannot accept any responsibility for fetal health during your pregnancy, your child's health upon or after birth, or your own health should any problems arise. Every pregnant woman has individual nutritional needs. While using the information in this book, you should consult with your obstetrician or public health nurse about the requirements of your individual condition.

Copyright © 1994 Sharon K. Yntema

Book and cover design by Mary A. Scott
Cover photograph by Nick Elias
Illustrations by William H. Benson

Library of Congress Cataloging-in-Publication Data

Yntema, Sharon, 1951-
    Vegetarian pregnancy : the definitive nutritional guide to having a healthy baby / Sharon Yntema ; illustrated by William H. Benson.
      p.   cm.
    Includes bibliographical references and index.
    ISBN 0-935526-21-8 : $12.95
    1. Pregnancy--Nutritional aspects. 2. Vegetarianism. I. Title.
RG559.Y58   1994
618.2'4--dc20
                                   94-8073
                                      CIP

This book is distributed to the book trade by Atrium Publishers Group, 3356 Coffey Lane, Santa Rosa, CA 95403. Please write for their most recent catalog, which includes all McBooks Press titles. Individuals may order this book through bookstores or directly from McBooks Press, 908 Steam Mill Road, Ithaca, NY 14850. Please include $2.00 postage and handling with mail orders. New York state residents must add 8% sales tax. McBooks Press publications can also be ordered by telephone from an independent book ordering service at 1-800-356-9315.

Printed in the United States of America

9 8 7 6 5 4 3 2

Contents

Acknowledgments

The author would like most of all to thank the many vegetarian mothers who contributed to *Vegetarian Pregnancy*. Their kind words and inspiring stories made this book possible. A special thank you is also due to McBooks Press, particularly to Alex Skutt for his ongoing support, to S. K. List, whose editorial assistance was painless and enjoyable, to Wendy Skinner for her skillful copy editing, to Kathryn Torgeson for her thorough indexing, and to Mary Scott for her careful design work. Thank you also to my family: to Billy for giving me the time, space and computer expertise to write this book, and to Niko for his encouragement and thoughtful comments at the times when I got stuck.

Introduction

In 1977, I was an idealistic vegetarian who became pregnant on purpose at the age of 26. In those days, vegetarian cookbooks struck average Americans as somewhat radical, and the healthiness of a vegetarian diet or whether vegetarians could get enough protein to survive were sometimes the subjects of raging debate among nutrition researchers.

Today, we probably hear more heated arguments over the extent to which meat and meat products are bad for our health. Doctors *have* reported cases in which a little meat appeared to make a particular person healthier. A majority of doctors nevertheless agree that most people would be healthier if they ate less meat. Without question, a diet based on plant foods rather than meat is now established as healthier, even as the fine points are still debated.

Plant foods offer nutritional protection against a host of ills—from high cholesterol to cancer. No one disagrees with this anymore, as the explosion of the health food industry demonstrates. As for the meat industry, a cartoon reprinted recently in *World Press Review* showed a loin of beef cut into its various drawbacks: steroids, colon cancer, growth hormones, pesticides, rain forest destruction, soil erosion, heart attacks, methane/global warming, herbicides, antibiotics and strokes. No one can ignore the dangers of meat, especially in view of the ways it is commercially produced for nationwide consumption.

In a recent issue of *Natural Health* (formerly the *East/West Journal*), a book reviewer of the newly updated 15th-anniversary edition of the *Moosewood Cookbook*, wondered, "It's lighter and leaner, but how's the taste?" The cookbook's author, Molly Katzen, rewrote many of her original recipes and the review compared the revised recipes and the old ones side-by-side. The new instructions replace richer dairy products, such as butter, eggs and cream, with foods lighter in fats, oils and calories, such as low-fat milk and yogurt. Although the reviewer recommended that the original recipes remain in print (with a wry suggestion for the alternate title "*Moosewood Classic*"), his testers for the most part preferred the lighter and sometimes spicier new recipes.

In the past, vegetarian cookbooks regularly included dairy-rich recipes to assuage the fear that, sooner or later, vegetarians were sure to expire from a lack of protein. Today plant foods are known to provide a very healthy diet, sufficient in protein as long as it is sufficient in calories. Recipes are now analyzed for fat and cholesterol content, and not only among vegetarians. "Light" cooking tips fill the magazines on supermarket racks, and a change in what our taste buds crave has occurred on a national level. Although the eating habits of most people are far from ideal, the number of consumer publications and the availability of products have expanded in all but the most remote areas of the United States. Most supermarkets carry tofu, a variety of vegetable greens and a selection of dried legumes. Increased interest in ethnic foods of all kinds has also focused attention on the foods of countries which traditionally have vegetarian cultures.

Concerns about good nutrition during pregnancy have also changed. These days, a doctor is more likely to know that vegetarianism is a healthy alternative, even without being sure exactly what vegetarians eat. Nutritionists are now commonly taught about scientific research that affirms the health benefits of a balanced vegetarian diet.

As a result, you are more likely to find doctors and nutritionists who will approve of your vegetarian pregnancy. But unless they specialize in vegetarian health, they will not have all the answers you may need.

Vegetarian Pregnancy is intended to help you find this additional information. It provides personal glimpses of true-life experiences of other vegetarian mothers, and it is also a source of cross-referenced information on nutrition and specific concerns of pregnant women. This material is designed to give expectant mothers practical suggestions from the research connecting nutrition and pregnancy. The approach is completely vegetarian, disregarding meat as a solution.

To use this book, I would suggest reading Chapters One and Two straight through. The first chapter discusses the question "Why have a *vegetarian* pregnancy?" I did not think of my own pregnancy as specifically "vegetarian," but I had to confront the same issues that arise for women who do think of their experience that way. I kept a diary while I was pregnant, as many women do, and found that a clear majority of the references were to food!

My own experience is only one of many, and Chapter Two is an inspiring collection of essays by other women. To compile this invaluable resource, I placed an ad in several magazines *(East-West Journal, Vegetarian Times, Mothering)* and had an excellent response. Although a lot of women didn't have access in their communities to all the nutritional information they needed, without exception, their vegetarian pregnancy experiences were positive. I have received some follow-up letters from women who wrote as mothers-to-be and have since had very healthy babies and feel great themselves. Some women (including me) had caesareans, but that does not have a nutritional connection, except in recovery, when good nutrition in a hospital setting becomes essential in returning strength to the body.

Chapter Three, focusing on concerns during vegetarian pregnancy, and Chapter Four, covering nutrients for a vegetarian pregnancy, could be read through, but are meant to be used for reference. Entries discussed under "Common Concerns" are listed at the beginning of that chapter; if you can't find a listing that matches your concern, be sure to look in the index. The concerns are alphabetized and cross-referenced with each other and with the entries in the "Understanding Nutrients" chapter, so you can pursue related nutritional concerns. If you have a concern which isn't listed in the text or in the index, let me know—I'll try to include it in the next edition. Write to: Sharon K. Yntema, PO Box 6879, Ithaca, New York 14851; no phone calls, please.

In the information presented, you will find that I don't dictate what to do. There is no one right answer to the supplement question, for example, because different people have different diets and individual nutritional needs. However, in *Vegetarian Pregnancy,* you will find at least as much and often more information than most doctors have to give you, along with the wisdom of personal experiences that can help guide you in making decisions.

In putting together this information, I hope that each woman who reads it will have the healthiest of pregnancies: a vegetarian pregnancy.

Chapter One

Why Have a Vegetarian Pregnancy?

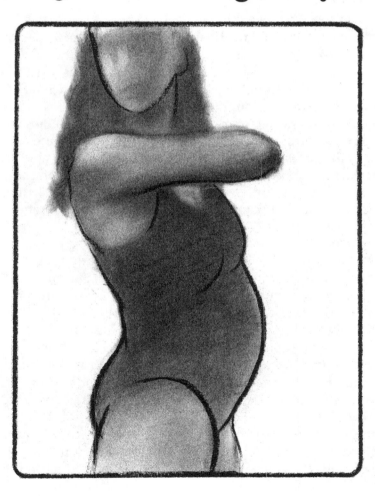

Whichen my pregnancy began, I had been a vegetarian for almost 10 years, and my husband had been a vegetarian for almost five. We lived in a city where being a vegetarian was practically considered normal. Our closest friends were not vegetarian, but since they liked bean tacos as much as we did, the difference in our diets was never really a focus at our weekly dinners together. If anything, they respected our choice for its health benefits. At Thanksgiving, we ate dinner with friends and various relatives and I always made a vegetarian main dish for myself and any other vegetarians on hand. It was never a "weird" recipe—usually stuffed squash or stuffed potatoes, something that looked familiar to almost everyone.

We belonged to a city-wide natural foods co-op and every week we were able to buy fresh organic produce, grown locally (within a 100-mile radius). Going to the Saturday food pick-up was a community event for at least a thousand people, so we never felt alone or strange in our eating habits, which were far from radical or fanatical in any way. My husband and I ate conventional vegetarian fare: lots of legumes and rice, with occasional eggs and milk. We believed brown rice to be an ideal grain and didn't use less familiar grains such as millet or bulgur until after our son was born. We rarely ate tofu or other soy products; our taste buds had not been exposed to them early enough and we could never quite enjoy them. Neither of us really liked milk or milk products such as yogurt or cottage cheese, so most of our dairy consumption was in occasional casseroles. I loved legumes with a passion and preferred fruits to vegetables, often needing urging to eat a daily salad. We had many favorite dishes to please our palates and we were both healthy. We felt so sure of the healthiness of a vegetarian diet that it did not occur to us to question it when we started on the road to being parents.

As it turned out, my vegetarian pregnancy was wonderful! I felt healthy, and after the first three months, I felt strong. The migraine headaches that I had suffered frequently for over three years vanished, as if by magic, relieving my worst concern: that I would need a prescription drug for migraine pain while I was pregnant. Since then, I have learned that the disappearance of migraines is a common side effect of pregnancy; as hormone levels rise, they naturally combat the trigger mechanisms of this devastating kind of headache.

Although I had avoided it for years, I started drinking milk again regularly, because I had been convinced by my parents that drinking milk was like an insurance policy. I didn't drink chocolate milk or drink milk with desserts, though, because I had heard that chocolate and sugar inhibit calcium absorption. I wanted the milk I was able to drink to go as far as it could nutritionally.

I was also worried about my nutritional vice—Coca-Cola—and whether I could give it up while I was pregnant. Once again, natural processes took over, and Coca-Cola started tasting bad to me. It is now common knowledge that pregnant women develop aversions to caffeinated drinks during pregnancy. At the time, I just felt lucky.

Tacos, one of my favorite meals, started to taste bad too. The beans and the hot sauce were unappealing for the first trimester, but my interest in them resumed during the second three months of my pregnancy. My doctor was sympathetic to a vegetarian diet and treated it as no big deal. He prescribed four supplements: a multi-vitamin/mineral

(Thera-M), iron (Org Iron), folic acid and vitamin E. I took the supplements without question, partly because I knew I wasn't eating very well during the first trimester due to changes in my appetite. Once my appetite revived, I felt they were probably unnecessary but I wasn't really sure. Most of my vegetarian friends took vitamins regularly, so I figured supplements wouldn't hurt and my body would excrete any excesses.

I felt noticeably weaker than usual during the first three months of my pregnancy, although I did not have any signs of morning sickness. My mother had experienced no morning sickness during any of her four pregnancies so, at the time, I felt that I had inherited her genetic tendency. In fact, I don't think such a link has been established yet. The weakness I felt was in my muscles and energy level—even doing simple, slow yoga exercises made me feel exhausted beyond belief. By the second trimester, this situation improved; I got my energy back.

After my first visit to him, my doctor sent me to the hospital for tests; these showed that my red blood cell count was good, and my urine had no signs of protein or sugar. This indicated to us both that my health was good and that I was at low risk for toxemia or anemia. I was assured that my appetite would come back and I was instructed to "eat to appetite," especially because, before pregnancy, I was a little underweight for my height. I was encouraged to gain 25 to 30 pounds, even though many other doctors of the time believed that weight gain should be more restricted during pregnancy.

At the time, an older co-worker boasted that she even *lost* weight during one of her four pregnancies and argued strongly in favor of minimal weight gain. I was glad that my doctor was from the new school of thought because I liked the idea of eating to appetite, trusting my body's instincts. Research now promotes a gain of 25 to 30 pounds for maximum fetal development and health. But at that time, it was difficult to accept the thought that a woman I respected deeply felt I was doing my body harm as she watched me steadily put on weight.

During the second trimester, I went from unsnapped jeans to looking undoubtedly pregnant. At conception, I weighed 119 pounds and by six months, I weighed 140. My waist went from 25 inches to 41 inches; my chest grew 3½ inches, and my hips expanded by 2 inches. I began to feel the weight of my breasts and felt as though I was waddling when I walked. But everyone I saw on the street showed me a feeling of good will that continued through the entire pregnancy.

My midwife asked me to record everything I ate for a week. This made me conscious that I didn't eat enough salads. I had braces on my teeth during my pregnancy and found salads very hard to eat, because the little pieces of raw vegetables would take forever to clean out. But I usually ate a salad every day, keeping in mind how important it was for the baby inside me to get those nutrients.

At about five months into my pregnancy, I experienced heartburn for the first time. I learned quickly that I had to eat less, but more frequently. I was able to help prevent indigestion by taking a few slow, deep breaths before meals, keeping my throat elongated by pointing my chin up in the air while I relaxed. This helped to calm down any immediate tensions which might have increased stomach churning.

During the fifth month, I also got a charley horse—a muscle cramp—in my right calf. It woke me up at night and I writhed in pain, fighting it with my whole body. It occurred to me that childbirth might be similarly painful and I should see this as a practice lesson, so I started trying to relax my body and to breathe deeply and regularly. The cramp went away, but my leg ached the next day. I wasn't sure I wanted to have that kind of practice again, so I followed Adele Davis's advice to increase my calcium and vitamin B_6 intake. Since processed milk has so much phosphorus, also implicated in leg cramps, I turned instead to calcium pills that included magnesium with vitamin D. For a snack one day, I recorded having two peanut butter/honey/wheat germ sandwiches, along with the following supplements: 595 mg of potassium gluconate, 50 mg of vitamin B_6, and 540 mg of calcium with 330 mg of magnesium.

I didn't have leg cramps again for another month and I reduced the supplements. But then one night I was rudely awakened by a double whammy—cramps in both calves of my legs. However, I reacted quickly, by breathing deeply and relaxing immediately. I remembered not to point my toes, but to flatten my feet as if I were standing. This time, the cramps disappeared very quickly.

My rate of weight gain had slowed by the seventh month, when I gained only 2½ pounds. My urine was showing a trace of protein, but my blood pressure was still low and I had no signs of edema (swelling), so the midwife and doctor were not worried. But at the end of my seventh month, the doctor found a little fluid retention in my ankles and told me to reduce my salt intake. This was difficult since I really like the taste of salt and couldn't believe it could be hurting me. I was very depressed after that visit with the doctor, feeling that what was *really* good for me and what felt good were at odds and that I hadn't been living up to the responsibilities of my pregnancy. I wished that my husband could be the one carrying the baby because he would have a much easier time obeying all the rules. I compromised by cutting down on salt somewhat, but not completely. Since then I have learned that salt restriction is not a good response to edema.

My midwife had urged me to increase my protein intake, since I was showing traces of glucose in my urine and my blood pressure was going up and down. Protein is known to decrease the incidence of toxemia, of which I was showing preliminary signs. I ate as much protein as I could, which meant I constantly felt uncomfortably full. My weight was approaching 150, a gain of almost 30 pounds during pregnancy. My doctor and midwife felt this was okay, but it was reaching a high level, so they were keeping an eye on it.

On the night I went into labor, my blood pressure went sky-high (146/96) and the midwife said she would not feel safe doing a home birth. After nine months of planning to give birth at home, I was very disappointed, but soon I was at the hospital, with my husband and sister at my side. Despite heavy labor for the next six hours, my cervix did not dilate and at 9:58 the next morning, my son was born by cae-sarean, as far a cry from a home birth as we could have ever imagined! But he was healthy, at textbook average size: 7 pounds, 11 ounces, and 21 inches long.

As I write this book, I have a very healthy, smart, tall and handsome 14-year-old vegetarian son who weighs 120 pounds and is 5'9", taller than I am. At age two, he had chickenpox (and gave it to me) when it went around the day care center but, other than that, he has been healthy and active all his life. He has never tasted meat, he hasn't been to McDonald's, and he has never regretted it. Some of his friends eat meat: he no longer feels sorry for them, but he is oblivious to peer pressure on the subject. He just can't understand why anyone would want to chew on a piece of meat.

Studying the research and other literature on vegetarian children, I find that my son fits into a pattern that is emerging, now that information about vegetarian diets is more commonly available. His health and brain power are above average, something noted in other vegetarian children these days. He is taller than average, which is probably more a result of genetics than diet.

Best of all, every time I read about changes in nutritional guidelines, I am reassured: A vegetarian diet is now correlated with lower cholesterol, lowered risk of atherosclerosis and osteoporosis as well as heart disease in general. My son has had a vegetarian diet from the day of conception and, because of this, is far less likely to have health problems when he is older.

Of course, he's not the only healthy vegetarian child around. I have received letters from vegetarian parents all over North America (including Mexico, Canada and Alaska, as well as Hawaii) who have had similar experiences. In general, my conversations and correspondence with vegetarian mothers suggest they plan their pregnancies ahead of time. They may approach pregnancy wondering if their diet will support the growth of a healthy baby, but they are usually confident of their own health, a crucial first step.

Before long, the principles of a truly healthy diet, which include decreasing meat products and increasing plant products, will be taught in schools, replacing the outdated "Four Food Groups" that most of us grew up with. The new food pyramid established by the U.S. Department of Agriculture in 1992 supports a vegetarian diet, putting meat and meat products into an optional category. Don't be surprised if this attitude becomes even stronger as nutritional research continues to confirm the health hazards of eating meat.

But here at the end of the 20th century, we are still in a period of transition. Even in this age of media, information presented in book form takes time to update. Any nutrition book which promotes choices based on the old "Four Food Groups" needs to be revised. Within the vegetarian community itself, the notion of protein complementing needs to be updated: carefully balancing plant proteins is not necessary to a healthy vegetarian diet. In the 25th-anniversary edition of her *Diet for a Small Planet*, Frances Moore Lappé clearly takes this position, admitting that her previous editions had produced a popular misconception that getting adequate protein on a vegetarian diet was difficult without paying attention to the amino acid content of each food.

We now know that eating a complex-carbohydrate plant food diet provides plenty of protein, as long as the carbohydrate intake is sufficient. In fact, in most recent writing about vegetarian concerns, getting enough protein is rarely the central issue. Instead, the emphasis is on eating whole grain meals and less dairy. Whole grains supply plenty of protein and are important because they provide the complete range of nutrients as well as taste satisfaction and appetite satiation. Increasingly, dairy products are seen to contain many of the same health dangers found in other animal products. Although the moral argument against eating dairy products may not be as strong as against eating meat, the health risks of high cholesterol and chemical contamination are just as pressing.

Even though current scientific research supports a vegetarian diet, it always takes time for new information to influence cultural habits. In the United States and other industrialized countries, diets are normally meat-centered. Most people find meals without meat strange and disorienting. While some vegetarians are able to live in communities where their food choices are respected, many pregnant vegetarians still find themselves viewed with suspicion when they talk to a doctor about their diet. Education is necessary. (References listed in the "Common Concerns: Social Pressure" section of this book might be of particular help in communicating with the medical profession.)

A pregnant vegetarian will find digestion easier than a pregnant meat-eater. During pregnancy, digestion changes dramatically. First, the process becomes more efficient, so a higher percentage of each nutrient is absorbed. Second, foods move through the digestive system more slowly, and nutrients remain in the system longer.

Meat takes a much longer time to digest than vegetable foods and is unlikely to be fully broken down, even with the extra time. With hours of sitting around in the stomach and intestines, meat begins to putrefy (sorry to be so vivid!), and discomfort from gas and constipation is far more likely. Eating fewer (or no) animal foods will be easier on your digestive system, especially during pregnancy.

Pregnant women all over the world have found that meat becomes particularly unpleasant to them in sight, odor and taste. This is true even for meat-eaters and, as with other common aversions of pregnancy, may be an innate protective mechanism. Meat has a higher chance of being rotten or diseased than other foods and perhaps the body knows it.

If you have been a vegetarian for at least a couple of years before becoming pregnant, you will be less likely to experience doubts about your diet because you will have seen that it can keep you healthy and strong over time. Your body takes a while to become used to any new diet. In switching from a meat-centered to a plant-centered diet, it will take time for your digestive system to clean itself out. Once you are used to eating grains and beans, the consistency of digestive juices changes to become much more efficient. For example, with a lower-protein diet, a greater percentage of calcium is absorbed, so less calcium is also required. During pregnancy, a balanced plant protein diet will provide plenty of both calcium and protein without overloading your digestive tract.

A 1990 report by the Institute of Medicine (part of the National Academy of Sciences, which determines the government's Recommended Dietary Allowance, or RDA) stated that complete vegetarians are more likely to have adequate nutrient intake of vitamin A during pregnancy than meat-eating women. Since vitamin A deficiencies have been linked to a higher rate of miscarriage, being a vegetarian has the built-in benefit of promoting full-term pregnancies.

This kind of nutritional protection is being discovered in many of the foods which are more likely to be eaten by vegetarians than those with a meat-centered diet. Other examples include the fiber content of fruits, vegetables and whole grains which aid in proper digestion (a prevalent concern during pregnancy) and vitamin C, which assists in iron absorption and strengthening the immune system. Vegetarians are less likely to have iron deficiencies during pregnancy than meat-eaters, as studies are now consistently reporting.

Protein intake is no longer considered a concern for vegetarians; rather, the health profession is now advocating a reduction in meat for all diets, because too much protein takes its toll on the human body, leaving systems clogged and slowed in efficiency. A high-protein diet tends to deplete calcium from the body as well, resulting in osteoporosis. During pregnancy, calcium levels are crucial to proper skeletal development of the fetus and so, once again, pregnant vegetarians have the health advantage.

According to recent reports, a deficiency of folic acid has been definitely linked to birth defects. Folic acid, which is found in raw green vegetables as well as legumes and whole grain breads and cereals, is lacking in most meat diets. Because meat is so packed with protein and fats, most meat-eaters don't add sufficient vegetables and whole grain foods to their regular diet. As a result, their diet is far less balanced and healthy than that of a vegetarian, who eats whole grain foods for their protein level, and vegetables as a central part of every meal.

Assurance of such advantages in a vegetarian diet during pregnancy rests on the presumption that the foods eaten are from a variety of plant sources, with a majority of carbohydrate intake coming from other than junk foods. In fact, if a pregnant vegetarian is getting sufficient carbohydrates from healthy sources, she is more likely to get sufficient quantities of the rest of the nutrients than other women.

Carbohydrate intake is now considered a primary concern: vegetarian women are likely to be thinner before pregnancy than is average for their weight. While a thinner body is often a positive sign during most of adult life, pregnancy and pre-pregnancy weight status are crucial factors in producing a full-size, full-term, healthy baby. Babies' low birth weight has been tied to both lower than average pre-pregnancy weight and inadequate weight gain in mothers. Since lower birth weight results in an increased risk of health problems and learning disabilities, sufficient carbohydrate intake is something pregnant vegetarians should pay attention to in their diets.

If you are a vegetarian, pregnancy is the time to fill up on whole grain muffins and breads rather than doughnuts and desserts. Snacking is encouraged during pregnancy, but raw vegetables and fruits—all you want—should be your choice, rather than candy bars and potato chips. By avoiding meat and meat products, you have taken an important step in giving your baby the healthiest possible start in life. But this *must* be complemented by a diet rich in vegetables, fruits and whole grain foods.

Pregnancy is a time when women experience a closer tie to their bodies and are more aware of their natural rhythms. The enhanced sensory awareness that comes with pregnancy is one preparation for the changes that are happening inside you. Because of the cravings and aversions that often accompany this, you may find yourself in a different relationship with food.

In my case, Coca-Cola suddenly started to taste bad and was simply no longer a temptation. On the other hand, my vegetarian diet had revolved strongly around beans and for a couple of months during early pregnancy, I did not want to look at beans, much less eat them, so I had to change the kinds of foods I ate. In retrospect, this made me vary my diet to a greater degree, something I'm sure was better for me and for the baby I carried inside.

What all mothers want most during pregnancy is the assurance that they are providing the best possible conditions for a growing baby. This may feel remote in the midst of morning sickness, but remember that your body pursues that goal on the biological level as well. During the first three months of pregnancy, a majority of women experience mild to severe nausea. As a result, we tend to pay a little more attention to our bodies, switch to a diet that is easier to digest and, best of all, give up many unhealthy habits: sudden aversion to caffeine, cigarettes and meat are common among women during this time. In effect, the body is purged without having to fast, which would be harsh and traumatic to a new pregnancy.

Throughout the first trimester, the embryo takes shape, changing from a single sperm and egg to a recognizable creature by its fourth month. The embryo is more strongly shielded from the external world during these first three months than during any other time. Using nutritional stores already in the mother's body, the fetus does not need a great deal of additional energy to grow during its first eight to ten weeks, so any nausea that cuts down on eating doesn't hinder fetal development. But to make sure these nutritional stores are available, it is important for a woman to be well-nourished before pregnancy begins. The nine months preceding conception are slowly coming to be recognized as equally important to a healthy pregnancy as the nine months after.

During the second trimester of pregnancy, the fetus is getting nutrition from the placenta which has been built during the first trimester, as well as a little bit directly from amniotic fluids. A mother's appetite often increases dramatically during her second trimester, in preparation for the last three months, when the baby grows so much that the placental stores cannot provide adequate nutrition: the mother must eat extra nutrients to replenish them. At that point, an increase in appetite is natural.

But even though you may be listening to your body's signals and making sure to eat well in response, those around you may not be so quick to understand and accept your diet. Knowing how to handle the changes of pregnancy in a vegetarian framework, and knowing that you are not alone in having a vegetarian pregnancy are additional ways to assure yourself that you are doing the right thing. Citing research will help reassure others, especially those in the medical profession. Telling the stories of other healthy vegetarian pregnancies will help reassure friends and well-meaning families to whom the idea is new.

Doctors and midwives may want to question you about specific nutrients, such as iron, folic acid, protein, carbohydrates and zinc. Concerns about protein are outdated, and you can be sure that anyone questioning you about this is not up on their vegetarian research. Iron, folic acid and zinc deficiencies are common during pregnancies, but vegetarians are less likely than others to have these problems. You have to remember that your doctors may still have to be educated and that friends and family may need to be reassured. And don't forget how important it is that you also have a gut feeling that what you are eating is good for you.

Here are some basic guidelines that can make your vegetarian pregnancy as healthy as it can possibly be.

1. Be healthy before you get pregnant. Although pregnancy usually inspires healthier eating and living habits as we try to nurture the new life within, the healthiest pregnancy starts before conception.

2. Once you are pregnant, take five or ten minutes a day to sit or lie down by yourself, with your feet up, in quiet comfort. Breathe slowly, without effort, and close your eyes. Try to become familiar with the way your body feels and senses in the moment. This simple grounding action will give you the chance to listen to your body. During pregnancy, body wisdom is very strong.

3. Keep a checklist of what you eat, aiming daily towards:
   • at least five servings of fruits and vegetables,
   • at least five servings of carbohydrates (whole grain foods preferred), and
   • at least two servings of protein foods.

4. Keep in touch with a midwife and/or doctor throughout pregnancy, from about the second month on. If an emergency should arise, it is important to be able to call on someone with medical knowledge of you as an individual.

5. Take it easy. Chew slowly and eat frequently for best digestion. Exercise gently throughout pregnancy. Take time

to grow a potted herb for your tea or greens for your salad. Relax while you watch the plants grow.

6. Trust your body and your appetite. Ask whatever questions you want or need to ask, especially of medical personnel. Remember that your body needs and rhythms will change throughout your pregnancy and that no one solution suits all people in all situations.

7. Know that a well-balanced vegetarian diet before and during pregnancy is the best gift you could give your growing baby. A healthy start is priceless and lasts a lifetime.

Chapter Two

Sharing Stories:
Vegetarian moms describe their experiences

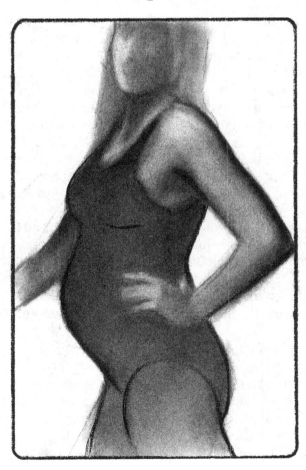

As I began this project, I placed requests for personal descriptions of vegetarian pregnancies in the pages of *East/West Journal, Mothering* and *Vegetarian Times*. The response was wonderful! About 150 women wrote to ask exactly what I was looking for. Some 75 mothers filled out a brief questionnaire, and about 50 responded in greater detail, sending everything from recipes to much more information than I could hope to use. From that wealth of material, I selected the following stories, with the goal of presenting both the variety and the similarity of experience in vegetarian pregnancies. I offer my deepest appreciation and gratitude to these mothers for their willingness to share their stories.

Regardless of its direction, no path is smooth all the time. But not a single person who wrote expressed any regrets about opting for a vegetarian pregnancy. Experience showed time and time again that fears over the nutritional value of a vegetarian diet during pregnancy were unfounded. One woman regretted the amount of milk she drank, and several others indicated they would like to reduce dairy and other lacto-ovo foods in their next pregnancy.

Some of the anecdotes in these stories speak to specific issues, so excerpts from them are repeated in the chapter on "Common Concerns." But the stories hold up on their own. They show how, given individual circumstances and approaches to diet, vegetarian moms and their families are making healthy choices and providing inspiration to all of us.

DEBORAH ALDRICH
Honolulu, Hawaii

Although life certainly is unpredictable, when I discovered I was pregnant, I made concerted attempts to control my own life and my baby's. That meant making important choices about what to eat and drink and how much to exercise. It wasn't until my first visit to my gynecologist that it ever occurred to me it might be unusual for a pregnant woman to be a vegetarian.

That day, Karen, a midwife working for the gynecologist, began what turned out to be a series of lectures on the dangers of vegetarianism during pregnancy. She was convinced that if I didn't follow the Federal Food and Drug Administration's recommendations for pregnant women, I was endangering the health of myself and my baby. That meant eating three servings of meat and four servings of milk every day.

"Why did you decide to become a vegetarian?" Karen asked.

"In the beginning it wasn't such a conscious choice," I answered. "I just didn't like meat. I was told that started about age one. I remember, throughout childhood, always drowning hamburgers and pork chops with ketchup to cover up the taste. As I grew up, I discovered a lot of good reasons not to eat meat, especially health and environmental reasons. For example, evidence shows that the less meat, dairy and eggs one eats, the longer and healthier life one has. And it is much more cost-effective to use land to grow vegetable foods than to grow grains to feed meat."

I don't know if Karen had expected such a lengthy response, but she didn't ask me to elaborate.

During my next visit, Karen exclaimed that the baby was coming along fine, that my heart was sound and my blood pressure was perfect. She then proceeded to share new information she had found concerning my vegetarian diet.

She'd even brought along a book about balancing proteins and amino acids.

I appreciated her concern, but I was certain that the nuts, grains, wide variety of fruits and vegetables I ate, as well as yogurt and cheese, were already supplying all the proteins I needed in the proper balance. I felt great and had already made it through the most crucial early stage of pregnancy without having any problems.

I was surprised when Karen continued to object strongly to a vegetarian diet during pregnancy, but she wasn't the only one. The mother of the two children I took care of said, "You can't be a vegetarian if you're pregnant!" It is such a common American misconception that one must eat meat in order to be healthy.

During my seventh month I had to give up riding my bicycle, because it became so awkward and exhausting. But then I got a job hauling newspapers around town. I got only about five hours of sleep a night, but I felt great. I was eating a high complex-carbohydrate diet which I felt kept me going strong all day. I ate almost continuously—whole grain cereals with soya milk, whole grain bread, vegetarian deli slices, salads, nuts, seeds, fruits, vegetables, cottage cheese, yogurt with a protein powder. . . . Every day was one big feast. Yet, I maintained a relatively low caloric intake and only gained 28 pounds by the time I gave birth. My son, Aaron, was born at 9 pounds, 4 ounces. When Karen popped in to visit the next day, I couldn't resist saying, while I held my busily nursing boy, "All of this, despite my vegetarianism." She smiled and nodded, still in disbelief, as she left.

NAOMI ARENS
Ballston Spa, New York

As a vegetarian, one becomes accustomed to friends, family, acquaintances and even total strangers offering unsolicited and—most often—conflicting nutritional advice. The questions are endless: How do you get enough protein? Do you take vitamins? What on earth do you eat? Don't you eat fish?

My husband is not a vegetarian, but he is very comfortable with my diet and loves the meatless meals I prepare. Before my pregnancy, we decided that we will raise our children as lacto-ovo vegetarians (a compromise, since he is a carnivore and, at the time, my diet was vegan). The only objection to this decision came from my mother-in-law, who commented that our child will be a "social outcast" if we do not allow her to eat meat! "What will you do when she's invited to a birthday party at McDonald's?" she asked. This really angered me. Why do meat-eaters place such importance on the social aspect of food? Besides which, I'd be a very fortunate parent if my greatest challenge in raising a child would be dealing with what my daughter eats at a birthday party!

For some reason, when I became pregnant, everyone and his brother decided I was incapable of making sensible food choices. Despite the fact that my obstetrician and pediatrician had no problem with my vegetarian diet, people were alarmed that I was not going to consume meat during my pregnancy. My maternal grandmother, who had never expressed any interest in my eating habits, called me in a state of panic during my first trimester. She had been convinced by some "very knowledgeable professionals" that if I did not consume meat during my pregnancy, then my baby's brain would be under-developed. The reason, she said, is that I would not be consuming any lysine. She urged me to please consider eating meat for the health of my baby, and would not listen to my reassurances that children of vegetarian parents are as healthy and intelligent (probably more so) than children of carnivores!

Even though I knew that my grandmother's friends were off-the-wall, my grandmother was genuinely concerned. I wanted to give her some factual information to reassure her, so I called the Vegetarian Resource Group in Baltimore, and spoke to their resident nutritionist. She told me that lysine is an amino acid, present in many common foods such as potatoes and corn. I also gathered up a few articles I found in *Vegetarian Times* and other vegetarian resources, and sent all this information to my grandmother. Apparently, she and her friends were still quite anxious for my baby's health, and are all so relieved now that Larisa is here and so obviously not lacking in health or mental ability. It is now a standing joke in my family that all our mental shortcomings are to be blamed on a lack of meat consumption!

TARA ASTOR
Mt. Holly, New Jersey

I am a 21-year-old college student with a nine-month-old son. I've been a vegetarian since I was 16. I had a relatively easy pregnancy, although Ian was 3½ weeks late. Even though almost no amniotic fluid was left, he came into the world (via caesarean) at 9 pounds, 8 ounces with an Apgar score of 8. He had no health problems whatsoever, even though the doctors weren't expecting a live baby!

Many of my friends were worried about my health while I was pregnant. My roommate from Texas (cattle country) warned me of how I was harming my child's health and my own as well. She firmly believes that one must eat meat in order to live.

I was going to a clinic in Florence, Italy, where I was studying at the time. My doctor really didn't seem concerned about me being a vegetarian. Italians aren't big meat eaters. I explained to her what I ate on a typical day: lots of whole wheat pasta, muesli, lentils, cheese, beans and huge amounts of veggies and fresh and dried fruit. She seemed quite impressed with my well-balanced diet.

When I came back to the States during my fifth month of pregnancy, I attended a clinic here in New Jersey. The nurse was always trying to get me to take an iron supplement. I was already taking Schiff's prenatal vitamins and I ate lots of iron-rich foods. My hemoglobin was never very high, but it never got below normal. I don't understand all the big hype about iron supplements. I believe in getting your nutrients from food.

The nurse also tried to give me some of their prenatal vitamins issued from the hospital pharmacy, the kind with the weird orange coating and God knows what kind of chemicals and artificial stuff inside. All they did was make me throw up, so I just stuck with the Schiff's vitamins.

Overall, I had a wonderful pregnancy, with no serious problems, except for Ian being so late. In fact, the only real problem I had being a pregnant vegetarian was getting good nutritious food in restaurants.

CECILIA KRUFT BARTLETT
Ontario, Canada

I have enjoyed two vegetarian pregnancies. I became a vegetarian when I was 16 years old, in 1969, for both health and spiritual reasons. I married in 1972, became pregnant for the first time in 1973, and gave birth to a beautiful, healthy, 7½ pound baby girl in April of 1974. Now, almost 20 years later, I'm still vegetarian, remarried and, at 39, pregnant once again.

I have remained in above-average good health over the years, getting most of my protein from a varied diet that includes soy and dairy products. I also take good organic and natural source vitamin and mineral supplements, which are more important than ever during pregnancy. I find that full-spectrum B complex gives energy and controls nausea, and 1,000 mg of calcium/magnesium helps control leg cramps. Vitamins C, E, D and iron are also important. I also try to drink several quarts of spring water daily. All these measures help insure vitality, calm nerves and clear skin. Fresh air and exercise are also important parts of my prenatal regimen, and a long daily walk (one to three miles) conditions the pelvic area, gives energy and promotes inner peace.

My daughter is now 18 years old and has been a vegetarian all her life. She is tall, with good bone structure, and has always been very healthy. She recently won a full scholarship to an Ivy League university. She says she has never craved a Big Mac. Neither have I, for that matter! I have not had any real food cravings during this pregnancy. I believe this is so because my diet is well-balanced and regular supplements and vitamins fill any other needs. I do drink a protein drink every day comprised of milk, yogurt, my favorite fresh fruits that are in season and protein powder.

I noticed that my appetite decreased significantly in my eighth and ninth month of pregnancy. As morning sickness faded away, I also felt less inclined to keep my stomach full. Additional pressure on my stomach from the baby growing inside may have helped. Or perhaps the summer heat just made it too hot to cook. A typical day's menu would be something like this:

Breakfast: fresh peaches, banana, strawberries, blueberries cut up into a bowl with milk (2 percent) or plain yogurt spooned over top and one piece of whole wheat toast.

Lunch: cheese, lettuce, tomato and sprouts sandwich on rye bread, glass of milk or spring water.

Dinner: huge salad of mixed greens with feta cheese and/or tofu and rice with steamed vegetables.

In my first vegetarian pregnancy, I drank lots of fresh-squeezed vegetable and fruit juices (celery/apple, carrot/celery and the like). In this pregnancy, however, I prefer to eat my vegetables and fruits whole and intact as a salad, for instance, because I find the increased fiber and bulk beneficial.

After my first vegetarian pregnancy in 1973-74, followed by a healthy, natural birth in a home environment, I gained great confidence. Here was living, breathing (and sometimes crying!) proof that it is possible, and desirable, to have a vegetarian pregnancy. I learned the value of commitment to one's ideals.

This time around, pregnant with my second child, I have no fears about my health or my baby's. I also know my recovery after the birth will be very quick. The strength of my convictions seems to fuel my physical strength of being.

The medical profession considered this pregnancy high risk because of "advanced maternal age." The doctors are hurriedly rewriting their opinions, however, because at 39 I have more energy and strength than most younger women, even those who aren't pregnant. My blood pressure is low and I have no edema. This is true, I am sure, because of my vegetarian diet.

My husband is also vegetarian, and I plan to have several more children in the next five years. We will raise them as vegetarians, too. I find that this diet and lifestyle teaches young children the value and sanctity of life. It also teaches them to make their own decisions and not to conform blindly. Vegetarian diet keeps one (at any age) calm and focused. This is very important and useful during the hormonal ups and downs of pregnancy. I received discouragement, negative questions and disapproval from family and doctors during my first vegetarian pregnancy. But most of my friends were also vegetarians at the time so I received lots of encouragement from my peers.

Now, after nearly 20 years, my family and new friends understand and respect my decision. Since all my medical tests look good with very healthy results, they have relaxed their pressure. People tend to fear what they don't understand, and they certainly don't want to admit to eating wrong all their lives! It makes my day to see my teenage daughter sporting a button that says, "Love Our Animal Friends, Don't Eat Them."

Pregnancy is a time of blossoming. Life is burgeoning within. Awareness of life, and its preciousness and value, colors my every moment. Vegetarianism, during this special time, becomes a natural outgrowth from and progression towards my inner awareness. With life all around me and within me, it becomes impossible to think in terms of taking an animal's life to eat. Only life can nurture life; energy begets energy, love becomes the beloved.

PAULA BORENSTEIN
Elizabeth, New Jersey

I was following a macrobiotic diet for about two years before I became pregnant with my first child. I decided it would be the best diet for me and my growing baby. My gynecologist prescribed a routine prenatal vitamin supplement, but I didn't take it.

I attended Bradley childbirth class and the instructor was at first skeptical that I could fulfill my protein and calcium requirements on a macrobiotic diet. I kept faithful track of what I ate as part of the class and added up my calcium and protein intake. I was getting at least enough, and sometimes a little extra. She never doubted my diet after that and I brought in recipes and samples of my cooking for others to try.

I occasionally strayed from my macrobiotic diet. I had half a cup of yogurt once or twice, some pizza when we traveled. I had a strong craving for fresh fruit and dried pears and ate lots of apples and dried fruit.

During my second pregnancy, I followed a vegan diet that was not strictly macrobiotic. During both my pregnancies, I was very, very hungry and ate and ate. I gained about 50 pounds the first time and nearly that the second. I felt great and everyone said I looked wonderful. The weight came off easily afterwards and my babies are both healthy.

GAYLE BRANDEIS
Riverside, California

I was in Bali when I discovered I was pregnant. I had been there for a month, exploring the island's vegan delights as well as the incredibly rich native culture. My appetite was immense, even in the wake of a harrowing bout of stomach ailments. I consumed oceans of peanut sauce, bushels of tropical fruit, skewer upon smoky skewer of tempeh satay. Certain food smells would turn my stomach, however, and I began to suspect I was pregnant. A hard-to-find test confirmed my instinct. The next morning, after two years as a vegan, I ordered eggs for breakfast.

I cannot really explain why I chose to begin eating eggs and dairy products again. I know it is perfectly possible to have a successful vegan pregnancy, but somehow it felt right to return to a lacto-ovo lifestyle. Perhaps I was influenced by subconscious connections, my mind linking egg with womb, milk with breast. Perhaps I didn't trust my personal vegan protein consumption. Whatever the cause, I'm grateful I trusted my intuition about my diet, for I had a glowingly healthy pregnancy.

When labor came, it hit long and hard. On the third sleepless day of contractions, my midwife recommended that I eat something to keep my energy level up. How appropriate that my husband fixed me scrambled eggs. The first food I consciously ate as an expectant mother heralded the end of my pregnancy as well. A psychic once told me that eggs are a "soul food" for me—they supposedly feed my spirit as well as my body. As I ate those eggs between contractions, I did feel more than fed. I felt sleek and whole as an egg, radiant as milk, while I waited for and welcomed the baby those foods helped create.

BETH CARBONELL
Williamston, Michigan

When I became pregnant I began to look for information about vegetarian pregnancy. I firmly believed that a vegetarian pregnancy was a healthy choice but I was willing to learn about any healthier choices I could make. Also, all the mainstream pregnancy books advised drinking milk, but I can't digest milk and I don't like yogurt, so I was especially seeking information about calcium intake.

Unfortunately, the only sources I had were my doctor and a vegetarian friend. The doctor was not too helpful. She recommended prenatal vitamins and tofu but I didn't find out until after my baby was born that she was also a vegetarian—I certainly could have used the support! The friend eats very differently than I do. She ate lots of yogurt, kefir, tofu and cheese during her pregnancy.

My husband and I base our diet on beans, vegetables, grains, cheese and fruit. We eat Mexican and Italian dishes, and hearty soups most of the time. We do not use food-combining, tofu or tempeh.

I finally gave up on outside information and decided to follow the messages my body gave me about what type of food it wanted. The first trimester was tough. We were remodeling the old farmhouse we had just moved into and it was summer, so I was living in the middle of a lot of dirt, chaos and heat.

I had nausea (it wasn't just *morning* sickness!) all day every day until month four and I even lost a few pounds. I craved nectarines, cold herbal tea and pizza. I don't think I ate much else that trimester. I was especially turned off by avocados and salad. If we cooked with garlic or onions, my husband had to cut and sauté them.

My appetite came back in the second trimester and I ate and ate. I wanted lots of vegetables, pasta, apples, cheese and chocolate. Late afternoon, which is usually my down time, I wanted chocolate the most. Evenings, after dinner, my husband would fix me cheese, crackers and apples. I ate about two apples a day. Strangely enough, I couldn't stand bananas, which I usually prefer over any other fruit.

I was gaining weight at a steady pace. My doctor was concerned that I might gain too much—she preferred her patients to gain about 25 pounds. Also, she ordered a few series of blood tests to be sure I didn't have any deficiencies. Upon receiving the results of these tests, I was quite pleased to hear that the news couldn't have been better. The doctor then pronounced me one of her healthiest patients. I was very happy to bring this news back to my non-vegetarian family!

During the end of the second trimester and through the third, I noticed a definite increase in cravings for sweets. I ate chocolate or ice cream every day. I seemed to want anything with lots of calories. Almost every morning I had eggs or French toast. I still had my pizza cravings.

During the third trimester, I started making hot chocolate in the evening. Although I could not drink cold milk straight, I could digest about 1½ cups of hot chocolate every day. My body seemed to need that or ice cream every day, as well as the cheese I ate most days.

I should mention here that I had terrible heartburn every single night during the third trimester. During the eighth and ninth months, I had to cut out my evening snack so I wouldn't have heartburn when I went to bed. I felt as if I were starving myself! Even a sip of water would keep me up at night. So, instead of eating at night, I would stock up on calories during the day.

What stands out in my mind about my pregnancy is that I had very definite cravings and dislikes. Whatever my body wanted I ate. I did not worry about cholesterol from the eggs or caffeine from the chocolate, or fat from the ice cream. This was my first full-term pregnancy after one miscarriage.

I'm usually very physically active, and I continued with walking and gentle exercise throughout my pregnancy. I'm average height and weight and I gained about 35 pounds during this pregnancy. Much to my family's surprise, I had a 9-pound, 4-ounce baby—no one in my family has ever had such a big baby!

After the birth I was a vegetarian nursing mama for eight months. I continued to eat what my body wanted. Within three weeks of the delivery, I lost all but 5 pounds of the weight. Those last 5 pounds didn't come off until 15 months of extra exercise later. Our son, now 16 months old, is a vegetarian. He is very healthy, very active, has never had an ear infection, and rarely gets colds. My son's doctor is not a vegetarian but is supportive of our lifestyle.

KIANA DICKER
Laveen, Arizona

As a lifelong vegetarian (even though I was force-fed meat by non-vegetarian parents for the first 16 years), I never doubted the healthiness of a vegetarian pregnancy. However, even the most stalwart and stubborn health food fan has doubts about diet fueled by the barrage of skepticism from friends, family and health professionals.

For myself, I caved in on the vitamin supplement question. I have a cupboard full of mineral and vitamin tablets which I normally use like medicine: C when colds are around, B for stress, multi when traveling, and so on. But, under the guidance of a sympathetic holistic doctor (herself the mother of two very young children), I dutifully downed a daily prenatal multi-vitamin pill.

After a week of stomachache and constipation, I put them aside, deciding to look closely at my diet and obtain appropriate nourishment from my food. Constipation is a common pitfall of pregnancy but I only suffered from it while ingesting the chemical vitamin tablets. Constipation is not a normal thing for vegetarians to experience.

My main focus, heightened by my mother's concern, was to eat enough protein. Although I try to go light on dairy products and eggs, I am a lacto-ovo vegetarian.

For breakfast I ate cereal with fruit, always including banana and juice and steering away from citrus because the acidity did turn my stomach at times. My one vice was one small cup of coffee with breakfast. I lunched on pasta or whole wheat sandwiches. And for supper I piled steamed vegetables, especially beets, cucumber, potatoes and broccoli, on a brown rice and beans base and doused well with lemon juice.

I went out of my way to eat whole foods and, although I succumbed to the odd pizza or two, I drove the extra miles to get fresh, organic food. I ate as well as I could without becoming a food fanatic, with all the stress that manic, obsessive behavior brings. I had a great appetite and blossomed from 106 pounds to a cuddly, rotund 145 pounds at delivery, most of which has fallen away without effort in the ten months since my daughter's birth.

I believe in letting the body tell you what it wants and then researching the validity of that desire. Throughout my pregnancy, increasingly, I lived with a greasy sensation in my mouth. I longed for licorice which, although normally good for women, can be an abortifacient for a pregnant one, and so I avoided it. This desire to freshen my muddy mouth then drove me to mint. I could down six boxes of Tic Tacs in one sitting—not good! Buckets of iced mint tea and chomping on mint leaves helped me avoid that. I also swathed myself in a highly aromatic aromatherapy cream. I really wanted to eat it, but smelling it calmed the irrational urge.

My inclination was to eat lightly and often, downing gallons of raspberry leaf tea and watered-down juices. Ginger tea and frequent handfuls of mixed nuts, dried fruit and figs banished all signs of morning sickness which had nagged at my peace of mind in the early months.

Concerned with consuming ample calcium, I loaded up with dairy products. I did not feel good drinking cow's milk. Goat cheese and soy milk felt better with the addition of a highly digestible calcium asporate tablet. Lots of liquids and dulse controlled the slight bloating which came during the second trimester. The last month I had nightly heartburn which was quelled with papaya, either fresh or tablets, and by munching anise and fennel seeds throughout the day. I boosted my iron intake with capsules of dock leaf and nettles—although I stopped this while nursing Sonora, since it made her colicky. My midwife recommended corn silk, which I took in a tincture, to flush the bladder.

Now, this is controversial, but I did drink alcohol during my pregnancy. A wine drinker, I sought an organic, sulphite-free wine and took one small glass with my evening meal two or three times a week. It helped aid my digestion, was relaxing and maintained a continuum in my social life which was wholesome and supportive. Although not a milk drinker, I found a couple of drops of tincture of skullcap and the smallest splash of whiskey in hot milk helped me sleep—an elusive thing in the last weeks of pregnancy when the hot Arizona nights and a big belly caused insomnia.

The only condition which I did not cure, but did quell, was work-related, a pregnancy-aggravated carpal tunnel syndrome. Wrist braces, a rice-based vitamin B complex, and exercise helped.

Staying physical, in tandem with truckloads of fresh fruit and vegetables (either juiced or whole), was the key to my health and positive attitude. I continued my usual workout until my body really began to change shape and then switched to Jane Fonda's pregnancy workout book and tape. I did a daily inverted yoga headstand and swam, swam, swam.

I really feel that taking control of my diet and herbal "medication" empowered me with the confidence to go for a midwife-assisted home birth. I stayed away from Chinese herbs because I could not research their use during pregnancy. With the exception of fresh parsley and watercress I dropped culinary herbs from my diet. My Bible was *Wise Woman Herbal for the Childbearing Year*, by Susun S. Weed.

I looked to plants for health and healing, for nutrition and medicine, and they did not fail me. Pregnant for the first time at 39, I had a happy pregnancy and an ecstatic childbirth, the latter aided by tinctures of motherwort, squaw vine leaves and blue and black cohosh.

Now ten months old, my daughter is on the right track developmentally and is exceptionally healthy (she's had only one cold) and fever-free. We communicated through visualization and meditation before birth and, born drug-free, she smiled before the umbilical cord was cut and has shown an alertness and awareness beyond her age.

CARMELA GUSTAFSON
Coram, New York

When I became pregnant with my first child in 1985, I had been vegetarian for ten years. The midwives who provided my prenatal care were aware of my diet but never questioned me about it, perhaps because my good health spoke well enough for its nutritional validity. Other than the common problem of a minor iron deficiency at about my fifth month (self-treated with an iron supplement), my pregnancy was trouble-free and I gave birth to a healthy 7-pound, 11-ounce baby boy. I went back to work part-time when he was eight weeks old and nursed him until he weaned himself two weeks before his fourth birthday.

Two years after that and still vegetarian, I had another healthy son who weighed in at 9 pounds, 11 ounces. Hospitalized for only 48 hours after a caesarean, I was home one day sooner than most women who have had vaginal deliveries. My second child is now nine months old and I have been vegetarian for a total of 17 years.

Looking back, I seem to have handled my vegetarian pregnancies in much the same way I first adopted the diet in 1975—that is, without much advance planning or conscious effort. When a friend, now my husband, told me he had become a vegetarian, the idea appealed to me almost on an instinctive level, as I had never before considered a change of diet. I gave up eating meat almost immediately, and did so without intending to make any social, spiritual or even nutritional statement.

So then, ten years a vegetarian and pregnant with my first child, I had kitchen shelves lined with Mason jars full of dried kidney, garbanzo and soy beans, lentils and split peas, kasha and barley, and brown, white and basmati rice. I had learned to cook with tofu, gluten and TVP; homemade breads and muffins rounded out the protein in my diet. I wondered why I was so often asked if I didn't miss meat, especially during my pregnancies. By then my diet had become a way of life and the foods I ate were the ones I craved.

Although I had given up on conscious protein complementing early on (it seemed to me that variety and good sense were all I needed to insure good nutrition), I found myself thinking about and seeking out proteins more often during my pregnancies than at other times.

For the first few months of my first pregnancy I drank a powdered protein shake for breakfast, but later found that regular hot cereals, pieces of fruit and cottage cheese, or even peanut butter served me equally well. When I felt a need to snack between meals (which was often), I ate raisins, peanuts, corn flakes, fresh fruit or chunks of cheddar cheese. I also allowed myself the luxury of eating as much ice cream for dessert as I wanted.

Since I tended to need lots of liquids during pregnancy and lactation with my first child, I satisfied this need primarily with milk and fruit juices, thinking these were healthier. With my second, however, I drank lots of water and juice and seltzer mixes instead and continue to do so while lactating. The nutritional outcome seemed to be the same and I gained 15 pounds less during my second pregnancy.

Although I ate more and at shorter intervals, my diet remained essentially unchanged while I was pregnant. I took multi-vitamins and an iron supplement, mostly as insurance against possible deficiencies during times when my appetite might have misinterpreted my needs. I felt strong and energetic throughout my pregnancies, worked and exercised through both until I gave birth, and had a positive outlook. I never had any serious doubts about vegetarianism in terms of nutrition and, by the time I became pregnant with my first child, I had been vegetarian long enough not to worry about whether it would be sufficient to satisfy increased nutritional demands. Over the years, I have collected a small library of vegetarian cookbooks, as well as non-vegetarian ones from which I glean or improvise meatless recipes.

Although I don't have the personality to promote actively the diet I embrace, I do pride myself on preparing varied, nutritious, satisfying and delicious meals without meat, poultry or fish. Family and old friends, none of whom are vegetarian, no longer ask what I could possibly find to eat beyond pasta and pizza. I am grateful to be enjoying excellent health, two strong and healthy children, and a diet which provides both satisfaction and inspiration.

MARIA JONAS INGBER
Philadelphia, Pennsylvania

My second suspicion that I might be pregnant introduced itself as I arrived late for work one day (oversleeping—my first suspicion) and headed for my requisite cup of coffee. Visions of a steaming mug of slightly sweetened java bounded in my brain.

My workday was usually fueled with a steady stream of caffeine coursing through my veins, but on this day Mother Nature had other intentions. As I neared the coffee maker, the brewed aroma assaulted my nostrils and sent me speeding for the ladies room. The mere thought sent my head (and stomach) reeling.

So commenced my first trimester, a good part of which was spent battling nausea. Feeling so sick jolted me; having been a vegetarian for five years I was used to feeling healthy, energetic and whole. I wondered if the constant queasiness was a possible flag that pregnancy and vegetarianism don't mix. Even friends and family thought it would be best if I returned to eating "normally."

Despite the doubts, my body demonstrated its worth glowingly. I couldn't tolerate anything containing caffeine, artificial sweeteners, additives or too much sugar. Physical exhaustion forced me to re-examine my crazy lifestyle and rest. I craved protein-rich foods (an area remiss in my diet) and, interestingly, pickled ginger (I recently learned that ginger is a natural "cure" for nausea). My body operated beautifully.

I embraced vegetarianism because it fit my beliefs; while I was pregnant, those same beliefs fostered a healthy, safe place for my baby to grow. A new-found respect for my body was my reward and my baby reaped the benefits.

STEPHANIE INGRAM
Greenville, North Carolina

I am a 26-year-old vegan who happens to be pregnant. There are many decisions I have made that are hard for some family, friends and health professionals to accept. The fact that I am happily single and not planning to marry has upset many people. My plan for a home birth has also been a source of conflict but, to my surprise, my diet has caused the most controversy.

I have been a vegetarian for eight years, having given up meat and eggs when I left home for college. Two years ago, I quit eating dairy completely. My reasons for being a vegetarian began with "cow love," but as I educated myself, I realized that ecological and personal health benefits reinforced my decision.

The people who question my diet and motives are for the most part well-meaning but, unfortunately, ignorant as well. They believe I need animal products to get protein, iron, calcium and other nutrients. Many say that I owe it to my baby to eat meat and take part in meat-eating rituals. I tell them that I owe my baby the safest chances for a healthy life, which is why I stay clear of drunk drivers, x-rays and animal foods.

At the local health department where I have been going for prenatal care, I exhaust the staff with my unending questions. I am the first vegan they have ever met there. The staff all like me and are intrigued by my choices, but also think I'm a little crazy to take a chance with a diet they know nothing about.

As part of the program at the health department, I [am scheduled to] speak with a nutritionist three times a week throughout my pregnancy. I sure threw that woman for a loop. She expressed her point of view, that cow's milk, eggs and at least a little bit of fish now and then are necessary during pregnancy. When I told her that fish is meat and that I don't drink of the cow, her face shot up from her stack of papers and she looked at me with shock.

I explained to her that I use soy and rice milks in my diet and that, like those with lactose intolerance, I don't eat cheese. The nutritionist had never heard of soy or rice milk, soy cheese or tofu ice cream. She was very alarmed when I told her I was drinking red raspberry leaf tea and asked me to stick to apple juice or some frozen concentrate.

I soon understood that the extent of her nutrition education was very limited. She believed in reading food labels to get a good diet. How unfortunate for women who have needs outside that!

My enjoyment and apparent health from eating an animal-free diet stunned and confused her. But as I was leaving her small office, she stopped me. She requested that I bring her a sample of my soy milk to my next visit. Happily, I agreed. The doctors and nurses have started to applaud my health status, attitude and interest in the whole baby experience. But even with my low body fat, low cholesterol, healthy lungs and heart, and sturdy build, they still worry that something is missing!

Frequently, my friends, many of whom have had their own babies recently, question me about my diet, wanting to know "the facts." Many of them were plagued with cravings, emotional fluctuations and excessive weight gain. As they laughed about the times they ate entire large pizzas with all the toppings in one sitting, I tell them than I've had only one craving, which was easily satisfied with a jar of artichoke hearts.

Despite the criticisms, I am doing quite well and feel I am on the right track. I've gained the right amount of weight, have no mood swings, nausea, or other common discomforts of pregnancy. Best of all, because I feel so healthy, I am sure what I am doing is best for me and the baby. I never have to feel guilty for what I put in my mouth, even when I indulge in an occasional cookie or other treat.

I believe that pregnant women who take care of themselves physically, emotionally and spiritually have less to worry about. The more we feel confident and healthy with less stress, the more our babies benefit.

Being a vegan has allowed me to view my baby as a wonderful bonus and not something that has turned my body upside-down. I don't have to alter my lifestyle or to worry about my every move. Best of all, my baby is getting a head start on a way of life it took me 18 years to discover. He or she will be brought up to respect all animal life, the ecological world as a whole, and his or her personal bodily health.

VIRGINIA IZQUIERDO
Dunedin, Florida

I have been a lacto-vegetarian for 20 years, my husband has been one for 18, my two sons, four and seven, since birth. My husband and I just turned 40.

When I was pregnant with my first child, I was thrilled, ate well, sang, danced, was very happy, read and prepared profusely. Unfortunately, I went to the hospital too soon after my water broke and was not even allowed to remain ambulatory. I was strapped down on my back and attached to a fetal monitor. I ended up with a caesarean that could have been avoided.

I wanted to have my second child at home, and was able to find a midwife to provide prenatal care. I normally weigh 110, but I gained 55 pounds during my second pregnancy, primarily in response to my midwife's concerns about my diet. Since she was not a vegetarian and I was, she was extremely concerned that I might not be getting enough protein to make a "healthy and normal" baby. She fretted about it a lot.

She told me that I had to drink the kind of protein powder drinks found in health stores three times a day, the kind recommended for body building—you know the kind I mean. Motivated by the desire to do the "right thing" and hoping that I could have my second baby at home, I followed her advice.

I had my second son by caesarean after 35 hours of labor. In retrospect, I'm convinced that if he had been smaller, I might have just popped him out squatting in my back yard. But he was 24 inches long and weighed 10 pounds. I'm convinced that gaining this kind of extra weight made the home birth impossible. With more information about a balanced vegetarian diet during pregnancy, perhaps things would have turned out differently and I could have had my baby at home.

DEVORAH L. KNAFF
Riverside, California

I never thought consciously about having a vegetarian pregnancy because I had already been a vegetarian for 14 years before I became pregnant. Asking me whether I would continue to be a vegetarian would have been like asking me if I intended continuing to wear clothes during my pregnancy. However, once I became pregnant, the issue of being a vegetarian came up in three different arenas: in my dealings with the medical establishment, with friends and family, and in my feelings toward my own body.

I had few problems with the medical establishment early on in my pregnancy simply because I didn't tell my doctor that I was a vegetarian. She told me to eat a healthy diet and I knew I was already doing that. However, during my third trimester, I was diagnosed with gestational diabetes—a diagnosis contradicted by several other tests. Nevertheless, after several of these tests, I was sent to a dietitian who gave me a standard meat-based diet to follow closely.

When I told her I was a lacto-ovo vegetarian, she first told me to "just go ahead and eat meat until the baby comes." Seeing me silent and aghast, she then suggested a series of alterations to the diet that left it almost entirely without protein. When I pointed this out, she answered that milk products and eggs were unhealthful because they contain fat and cholesterol and I should just have apple slices if I got hungry. At that point, and since all tests subsequent to the first one had proved negative, I simply listened quietly to her for the rest of the visit. I went home and threw out her diet, ate as I had before, and had no additional problems.

Less easily resolved was the way friends, acquaintances, and family members treated my vegetarian diet on a daily basis throughout all nine months. People I had known for years and who had ignored my eating habits suddenly displayed the urge to criticize me. "Are you *sure* you're getting enough protein/vitamins/calcium?" people frequently asked. One person actually said in dark tones, "Something might happen to the fetus and you would always have to wonder if your diet didn't have something to do with it."

I often felt something very close to rage at these comments, both because I knew my diet was much healthier than theirs or those of most pregnant women, and because I resented the fact that, as soon as a woman becomes pregnant, people feel quite free to treat her body and habits as public property, subject to public opinion. I tried to be courteous, a trait my Southern mother had bred into me, but during the last few months of my pregnancy I began telling people to leave me alone and that it was none of their business.

While my encounters as a pregnant vegetarian with both medical professionals and my intimates were often a cause of stress, being a vegetarian helped me significantly in the way I viewed my own body.

I had the kind of pregnancy that no one, not even my pregnancy books, really prepared me for. After three months of throwing up and constant nausea and dizziness, I waited for the morning sickness to stop. After five months, I was still waiting. At about six months, I was still constantly nauseated—it was like being car sick for months on end—but the dizziness was gone. At seven months it was back and I started vomiting even more.

The symptoms of "morning" sickness finally disappeared about halfway through labor. I remembered thinking a moment after I had given birth to my daughter, that the most wonderful part of giving birth was not the cessation of pain, but the fact that I wasn't nauseous anymore.

As a result of being so thoroughly sick the entire pregnancy, I never had the weird food cravings that have been fodder for stand-up comics for years. I never wanted food at all and, for the first time in my life, began to have an antagonistic relationship with food, a relationship that might have been a metaphor for the way I felt about my pregnant body. I knew that pregnancy might not be entirely pleasant, but I did expect to enjoy some of it.

One day, as I was boiling some spinach, which was the only possibly palatable thing at the moment, I suddenly saw food—that is to say, my commitment to being a vegetarian—as central to getting me through the difficulties of pregnancy. Not only, of course, did I need the calories and nutrition of food, but the principles that led me to become a vegetarian—the principles of respecting and valuing other animals too much to eat them—were a core of my strength, a strength that got me through months of lying on the bathroom floor for hours every morning.

After that shift in perspective, which happened during my fifth month of pregnancy, I began to visualize what food I could get down as a contribution both to my daughter-to-be's physical strength as well as her moral fiber. I could feel my baby growing strong on the fruits of the earth, not on the pain of other sentient creatures.

For now, my two-year-old daughter is happy with her vegetarian diet. Our household is vegetarian in orientation although her father still eats meat. I am enjoying this peaceful period before she goes out into the world on her own, a place where her friends may have hot dogs and cheeseburgers while, at home, we do not.

MONICA LEAL
Converse, Texas

My story actually begins seven years before I became pregnant. At the age of 20 I was diagnosed as having endometriosis and was told I would probably never be able to get pregnant unless I underwent major surgery. I did not have the surgery but instead sought alternative methods of healing. I went through a detoxification program which included colon cleansing, mega-vitamin therapy, and drastic dietary changes. With the guidance of a nutritionist, I began eating more wholesome foods and cut out all junk foods. Although the nutritionist was not a vegetarian, she believed dairy products were mucus-producing, so I cut out all dairy products as well. Within a few months my menstrual problems began to clear up and so did my sinuses. My health had already improved so much that, when I read some vegetarian literature, I decided to take it a step further and made the commitment to vegetarianism.

Upon giving up all foods that once had a face, I felt an even higher level of energy and clarity. Over the next six years I maintained a 100 percent vegetarian, 99 percent vegan diet (I never ate eggs, and I found I could tolerate a little cheese only occasionally—more than once or twice a month would give me sinus headaches again). Colds and flus would be going around at work, but I just didn't get sick, whereas before I was sick quite often.

During those years, I learned that even so-called "natural" vitamins are chemicals and are not recognized as food by the body. I began to phase out vitamins and got more into herbs and "super-foods" such as bee pollen, royal jelly and blue-green algae. The blue-green algae, in particular, seemed to boost my health dramatically. Diet and herbs had regulated my periods, but I still had some PMS symptoms until I started taking the algae. I believe this is because it supplied the trace minerals missing in everyone's diet, vegetarian or not. I also began exercising regularly so, by the time I had gotten married and was ready to start a family, I felt certain that I would have no trouble getting pregnant. And I didn't. I got pregnant right away! My husband and I were elated!

By this time, I believed in vegetarianism so strongly that there was never any doubt that it was the healthiest diet for any time, including my pregnancy. However, all of the books I had at the time, which were my only source of support, dealt with lacto-ovo vegetarians, not vegans. I was concerned about calcium and simply did not have the knowledge of how to obtain enough calcium on a vegan diet while pregnant. I decided to err on the side of excess and drank huge amounts of raw, certified goat's milk throughout the pregnancy.

Big mistake! Although goat's milk is more assimilable and less mucus-producing than pasteurized cow's milk, it is extremely high in fat. I knew this at the time but figured I wouldn't have any trouble losing the weight later.

Wrong! I gained 20 pounds more than I was supposed to and three years later still have not taken it off. Keep in mind that I exercised regularly (five times per week) during my pregnancy and have continued to do so since. I never touch ice cream, butter, sodas or any of those other dietary "evils." I do believe goat's milk was the culprit.

I want to cleanse my body and lose weight before I get pregnant again. I am currently going through a cleansing process and have found an accumulation of mucus in my system. I don't think I absorbed the calcium in the goat's milk very well, because after my baby was born my teeth looked worse. I do not plan to repeat this mistake with my next pregnancy. I have discovered more information relating to vegans and now have the confidence to remain true to my vegan self.

In fact, I am gravitating in the direction of a diet composed primarily of raw foods and I believe I will continue this throughout my next pregnancy. Such a diet includes large amounts of freshly extracted vegetable juices, including an abundance of green juices, as well as a variety of sprouts, nuts, seeds, and nut and seed milks. I will continue to include such staples as tofu, tempeh, whole grains, legumes and so on, which are cooked, but I am definitely in the process of increasing the *proportion* of raw foods in my diet. I have come to the conclusion that such a diet will not only be adequate for pregnancy but will probably be closer to optimal.

Another mistake I made during my first pregnancy was stuffing myself with protein. Now, of course, I am aware that protein needs increase during pregnancy, but I think I overdid it. I had been dismayed to learn from a nutritionist friend that, yes, the protein charts were correct, and I was so concerned about doing everything "right" that I literally snacked all day—even when I wasn't hungry—on wholesome, high-protein vegetarian foods, counting protein grams all the while. I did not take into consideration, however, whether or not I was actually assimilating all that protein. I definitely should have eaten more salads and other raw veggies to help digest the protein. I have since learned that protein consumed in its raw state has enzymes and is more assimilable, and therefore less of it is needed. I think next time I will concentrate more on raw protein sources such as sprouted legumes, soaked seeds, nut milks and so on. I think I will also be more attuned to my body's needs rather than blindly following charts. Charts are important, of course, but it's also important to listen to one's body (provided the body's signals are not being distorted by junk food addictions).

Overall, however, I believe my diet was very good during my first pregnancy. I never took an iron supplement but maintained a high level of iron just from herbal teas and blue-green algae. I felt great through my pregnancy and never had any morning sickness, constipation, hemorrhoids, high blood pressure or any of those other problems commonly associated with pregnancy. In fact, two acupuncturists separately told me that I was very healthy and they could barely find anything to do with me!

My son is now 3½ years old. He was totally breast-fed and has never tasted any meat at all. He's never tasted candy either, nor any other sugary snacks. I give him treats, but they are whole grain, honey- or maple-sweetened. This child has never been to a doctor because of an illness; I have taken him only for well-baby checkups. He has never had an ear infection or a very high fever. The few colds he has had were mild and responded quickly to herbal treatment. I have observed that his worst colds have usually been shortly after consumption of cheese. To us, dairy cheese is a treat, to be indulged in only occasionally, such as the cheese pizza at birthday parties. My son does not drink cow's milk or sodas, nor does he eat eggs. His skin feels like silk and he is beautiful, strong and full of energy. He is living proof that a whole-foods vegetarian diet is optimal for pregnant women and for children.

FAYE LILYERD
St. Paul, Minnesota

My husband and I adopted the "Fit for Life" eating style in 1987, after reading the books written by Harvey and Marilyn Diamond. On average, I ate fruit until noon, a salad for lunch, and heavier foods at supper. I was also drinking a fresh glass of carrot-apple-beet juice in the morning, until I realized I was two months pregnant.

Light morning sickness started at that time and I couldn't keep juice down. The sight of fruit made me nauseous. I ate cereal and toast for breakfast, using nut milks and soymilk. Fresh vegetables still appealed to me. My nausea lasted only a month, but my tolerance for fruits stayed low, only about half of what I was used to.

In the third trimester, I craved breads, potatoes and pasta. Our birth instructor told me that insufficient protein intake could result in craving carbohydrates. I ate more raw nuts and tofu, which seemed to help. We are skeptical about consuming too much protein, even it if comes from non-animal sources. In a protein-obsessed society, it is hard to feel at ease eating small amounts of protein, even though our bodies require less than what is considered normal and function better that way.

I have a history of low iron. During pregnancy, I increased my intake of raisins, prunes, spinach and broccoli, and was able to raise my iron level.

Periodically, I questioned my vegetarian diet and pregnancy. My husband always assured me we were both okay and pulled out health and diet books for reinforcement. It also helped to have pregnant friends who were vegetarians when these doubts arose.

Our child was born, a full-term, healthy baby, perfect in all respects. The nurses commented on how alert and attentive he was from the start—I was so proud! We had had a wonderful pregnancy, complication- and medication-free labor and delivery, and a beautiful new baby—all with a vegetarian lifestyle.

DEBORAH MCGRATH
Lorton, Virginia

During the first trimester of my first pregnancy, I began to follow a vegetarian diet. The reason for the change in my diet was an increased awareness of my body due to the pregnancy, and the fact that I had begun to work as a book-keeper for a small chain of health food stores.

As my knowledge grew, so did my concern—not only for my own health, but also for the health of my child. I found that as I made changes in my diet, I could feel the benefits immediately. Common problems that most women experience, such as heartburn and constipation, were only experienced at the very end of pregnancy when the baby was very big.

I never experienced any food cravings either. My doctor's concerns were that I got enough protein in my diet and, since I was already not much of a milk drinker, that I wouldn't get enough calcium. I chose to use soy milk and I ate cheese for calcium. I also ate plenty of legumes to ensure protein intake.

At the recommendation of my doctor, I took a vitamin and mineral supplement which I had obtained from our health food store. I took them throughout the pregnancy and while nursing.

After the birth of my son, I decided to maintain this way of eating because I had never felt better. Since I was breast-feeding, the continued interest in my nutrition for the sake of my child was also a concern. Plus, I had found the flavor of fruits and vegetables organically grown much crisper and much more pleasing to my palate. Another bonus was losing my pregnancy weight quickly and easily, with my concentration primarily on toning exercises.

Following a vegetarian lifestyle became very comfortable for me and, when I discovered that I was pregnant with my second child the following year, I continued with it. I had no problems again this time. Since I was using the same obstetrician, he again reminded me of his minor concerns. I followed the pregnancy the same way I did the first, and the birth of my second child was almost as smooth as the first, except that it was a caesarean, and recovery was a little slower.

I continued with a vegetarian diet for myself and my children. I had by now gotten used to the taste of some products I had never previously used, such as tofu, soy milk and different cheeses, such as goat. I really enjoyed experimenting with different foods and recipes.

With my third pregnancy, the knowledge I gained during the previous years enabled me to make sound nutritional choices. At this point in time I became interested in macrobiotics. I had read a lot about it, and thought that the philosophy behind it was agreeable and made sense.

I began macrobiotics, and found many cookbooks and wonderful recipes to try. I did find, however, that some ingredients and foods were not always easy to obtain at the health food store or a local Oriental market. Luckily, with a little research I found an excellent mail order company where I could round out my shopping needs.

My doctor was concerned about this type of diet during pregnancy because a macrobiotic diet doesn't use soy milk or cheese. I did find a wonderful tea, which is a staple of the macrobiotic diet, called bancha. It is loaded with calcium, and can actually supply more calcium than dairy products, without the fat.

In the macrobiotic diet, vitamin supplements are not used either. However, after three months of following a strictly macrobiotic diet, I did stop and go back to a simple vegetarian diet. The health benefits of the macrobiotic way of eating are evident. But while my diet now incorporates a lot of macrobiotics into it, I have found that, for myself, it was too difficult to follow. It was hard too, to give up certain old favorites, such as honey and carob, especially when I still had to prepare meals for the rest of my family.

I still do love the bancha tea and many other foods I learned about through this diet, such as miso soup. This pregnancy and labor was the easiest of all three and I do believe that nutrition played a tremendous role. Through my experiences, I found that the most difficult thing involving my dietary choices during pregnancy were the opinions voiced by others, such as my doctor or family members who had never heard of a pregnant woman not drinking gallons of cow's milk. I was confident in my decisions, and knew I had carefully researched what vitamins and minerals a woman expecting should have in her diet. I am so happy with the changes I made years ago; I can't imagine going back to using meat and dairy products in my diet.

DEBRA NEWBY
Torrance, California

I took my 19-month-old son, Wesley, to the pediatrician for a checkup last week. After he examined the fish in the tank, opened all the cabinets and tangled up the curtains, we were seen by the doctor. The doctor examined my squirming son, and found that he was in the 90th percentile for both weight and height. The doctor then proceeded to ask me some questions. He asked me if I was giving my son whole milk yet. I replied, "No, he drinks soy milk."

The doctor then asked, "Is this by choice or because the child can not tolerate milk products?"

"This is by choice. We are vegetarians," I informed the doctor for the fifth time since my son was born.

The doctor then turned to write in his chart. He stopped and turned around. "Is Wesley vegetarian?!" he asked incredulously.

When I replied that he was, the doctor began rambling about the need for Wesley to have some blood tests and the need to check his iron levels. Then his voice trailed off. He looked down at my large energetic son who was trying to dismantle the chair and said, "Never mind. I think he is growing fine."

And he is growing fine. He has never had any animal products (except for honey). Though some of my friends worried about my decision to consume no animal products while I was pregnant and to keep my son on a pure vegan diet, when they look down at my happy child with his sparkling eyes and thick curly brown hair, they agree that he has not suffered for it. Instead, they make excuses about giving their own children meat, saying things like, "We're trying to cut back on how much meat we eat."

I became a vegetarian a few weeks before I conceived Wesley, my second child. I had just finished reading John Robbin's book, *Diet for a New America*, and decided that this was it! No more meat for me and my daughter Melissa. (She was almost two at the time.) For our family to retain its harmony and still incorporate my life-changing decision, I knew that I must also convince my husband. I informed him that I had a very important book for him to read, called *Diet for a New America*. He said he would some other day, but right now he was reading a novel. So I hid the novel and he read the book! He agreed that cutting meat from our diet was the responsible thing to do, both for our health and for ecological reasons. That was in January of 1990. I became a strict vegetarian; I consume no dairy products or eggs. My husband and daughter are vegetarian but still occasionally have cheese when they go out to dinner.

Becoming a vegetarian was very easy for me. It was almost a relief not to have to gag down meat any more in the name of getting "healthy protein." As I said, I became pregnant within a few weeks of making this decision. I had a very easy pregnancy. I never had morning sickness, and I had a lot of energy. (Well, until the very end!) I did not really have any cravings, but I enjoyed a large tofu, strawberry and banana shake almost every day. I did concentrate on eating a lot of vegetable protein, probably more than I really needed to.

I guess I still heard the voice of my doctor from my first pregnancy telling me to eat lots of protein (meat and eggs, of course) so that I would have a healthy baby. I added a lot of tofu and nut butters to my well-rounded diet of fruit, vegetables and grains. I began to collect vegetarian cookbooks and read everything about nutrition I could find. I found *Vegetarian Times* magazine to be a great resource. I never did tell my doctor about being vegetarian while pregnant. I realized that I probably knew more about nutrition than he did, and the consequences from this decision were my responsibility. Although once in a while I would doubt what I was doing (was I harming my unborn child?), most of the time I was content that I was giving my child the best start possible.

After nine fairly easy months, I labored at home for six hours and then went to the hospital for the final three hours. After a drug-free labor with no episiotomy or other medical intervention, I gave birth to a beautiful, healthy baby boy who was eagerly nursing within 15 minutes of his birth.

I know without a shadow of a doubt that I am doing the right thing in bringing my family up vegetarian. Both of my children are very healthy. Except for well-baby checks, we seldom see the doctor. In an age when multiple ear infections and ear tubes are common, both of my children have had only one ear infection each in their lives. So far, my children seem to be allergy-free, and they rarely catch colds. With the added milk hormones, contaminated meat and the pollution to land and water caused by the livestock industry, I don't see how a responsible parent could choose anything but a vegetarian diet for their children. How many kids say that artichokes and broccoli are their favorite food? Mine do!

JACKIE OLSON-NEWHOUSE
Austin, Texas

Because I had a history of poor health, my family and friends thought I was making a horrible mistake by choosing a vegetarian diet. It started when I met Christopher, a vegetarian chef who was very knowledgeable about nutrition. In the months following, I found I had never been so healthy in my life! I knew it had to be from the change in my diet: no more MSG riddled my head and, magically, headaches that I had been suffering for 14 years vanished.

I had also been anemic for years. When I started drinking beet juice, not only was I not anemic, but I suddenly had lots of energy. Up until that time, it seemed that the first thing on my mind when I woke up each morning was, "When can I squeeze in a nap?"

Of course, lot of friends and family refused to believe that a vegetarian diet could make me feel so much better, especially since western medicine never seemed to help me at all.

Later on that year, Christopher and I conceived our daughter. We felt that a vegetarian diet was the best choice for me for a healthy pregnancy. Now the heat was on. . . . Some of my dearest relatives started talking to their doctors about the choices I had made. I was bombarded with phone calls from them stating that the baby could not get the vitamins and minerals—not to mention protein—it needed if I continued my vegetarian diet.

Armed with facts, I tried to smooth things over, finally relying on the notion that "time will tell." After what I consider to be an easy pregnancy (good health and very little morning sickness), I gave birth to a beautiful 8-pound, 2½ ounce "vegetarian" baby girl at home, with the help of my husband, my mother, my twin sister and a girlfriend.

It has been a little over two years now. Our daughter Sophie is very energetic, curious and healthy. She has never eaten meat and will never find it served at our house. I know that one day she will want to try something that all the other kids are eating, but pray that with love, support and guidance, she will prefer the vegetarian lifestyle over pressure to be "normal."

SHARON OUTTEN
US Army APO, Germany

When my husband Steve and I decided to plan the conception of our child for the summer of 1991, we had no idea that Steve would be sent to war in the Persian Gulf just six months prior to our planned date. Though I didn't know for sure whether he would be coming back home alive, I decided to go ahead and prepare my body for pregnancy. I had been a vegetarian for a year and had been constantly educating myself in nutrition. With the help of a naturopathic doctor, I did a detoxification with herbs and psyllium hulls. My diet was very simple and fresh. I ate a wide variety of fresh, raw fruits and vegetables every day. I enjoyed plenty of whole grain products, beans, seeds and nuts, and I drank lots of soy milk, homemade juices, and worked full-time at a grocery store, took lots of walks, had a daily exercise routine, and made sure to take my vitamins regularly. During the entire six months of separation from my husband I was sick only once. Strep throat was going around my job and I began feeling sick, too. My doctor prescribed pure aloe vera gel, vitamin C, plenty of carrot juice and a few days of rest. I was back to work in no time! Soon after this, the war ended. Steve came home about a month-and-a-half later, just in time to conceive in the month we had planned!

Steve had just been stationed in Germany before the war broke out. Now it was time for me to go back to Germany with him. These first two months were the worst part of my pregnancy. Moving anywhere is always a little difficult. But moving to a foreign country and trying to find healthful places to eat while you're waiting for a refrigerator and all your furniture is downright nerve-wracking! There are plenty of places in Germany to get schnitzel, hamburgers, meat-laden pizza, soda and other unhealthy foods. But finding vegetarian restaurants, or even regular restaurants with healthful side dishes, is very difficult when you're new and don't know the language.

For the first two months, we ate poorly, consuming mostly processed foods. I experienced nausea, irritability and depression. Both Steve and I were feeling heavy, sick and constipated. The Army grocery store provided fresh fruits and vegetables, but there was not a wide variety and the quality was often poor.

With the exception of a few basic items, all the shelves in the store were filled with the normal denatured food-stuffs found in most grocery stores. It took a while before we found German "Naturkosts" and "Reformhauses" where we could get natural dried fruits, raw nuts, whole grains, soy products and other things we would normally find in a U.S. health food store. During this time, we ordered natural vit-amin supplements from the United States too. Our health and mood began to improve as our diet did. I bought yeast flakes from the Naturkost and my nausea began to subside significantly; after the B vitamins arrived from the States, it disappeared completely. In addition to eating right and tak-ing vitamin supplements, I made sure to take naps and to exercise daily. I was active all day, working at the post Burger King, and I took daily walks around the neighborhood. On weekends, Steve and I took three- or four-hour walks through the woods. The next seven months were absolutely beautiful.

I wasn't able to begin prenatal medical care until the third month of pregnancy. The two Army doctors I saw were very good and didn't treat me oddly because of my vegetar-ianism. I was truly surprised at that because I thought I would be hassled. Their feelings were that, as long as I was eating a wide variety of foods and taking my vitamins and iron, everything was just fine. I didn't tell them I was taking the natural vitamins that my doctor in the States recom-mended instead of theirs. As long as all my tests were com-ing out well, I saw no need to provoke trouble!

The feelings of family members were not exactly the same as my doctors'. Steve's side was sort of worried that the baby might come out malnourished or sickly. We weren't really aware of their feelings until after the baby was born. My side was a little more easygoing. They considered me to be slightly weird, but figured I had enough sense not to damage my child.

Our new Army friends were more or less curious. Many were couples who were expecting babies around the same time that we were. At first most of them felt that we were a little nutty! We never preached to them. As the months passed, they began to notice the differences in our pregnancies and that's when they began to ask a lot of questions.

Many were surprised that I didn't have leg cramps since I drank almost no milk and ate little of other dairy products. I explained that I drank freshly made carrot juice almost daily during the last trimester, much as they drank milk daily. They were surprised to learn how much calcium carrots and other vegetables contain. My boss and co-workers were truly amazed at my endurance and cheerfulness. I worked from my third month until two weeks before our baby was born. During that time I won three awards for service and customer friendliness. I don't know what their opinion towards vegetarianism was when I began working there, but everyone gained more respect for it by the time I left to begin preparing for our baby's arrival.

I must say that labor and delivery were all that Steve and I prayed it would be. The combination of proper diet, exercise, rest and super support from Steve helped everything go well. When we went to the hospital, we were expecting to be sent back home for false labor. Instead it turned out that I was seven centimeters dilated! I couldn't believe it and neither did the nurses.

Steve and I breathed, sang and laughed our way to the birth of our beautiful daughter, Jae. It was a lot of hard work, for sure. But it was nothing like the horror stories that many first-time parents are told. There was no screaming, cursing, punching or uncontrollable desire to pulverize my husband, just a lot of breathing and pushing. I didn't have medications or an episiotomy. I was 155 pounds when I went into labor. Jae was born at 6 pounds, 9 ounces. Now, five months later, she is a 17-pound bundle of giggles with two teeth. I am back to 125 pounds, thanks to nursing. After months of weaning ourselves from dairy products and reading various books on nutrition, Steve and I are now vegan. Our families have gotten pictures of Jae and are more comfortable now with our diet. To quote Steve's mom, "She's so fat! She's the fattest of all my grandchildren. All of them should be vegetarians!" Well, maybe, maybe not. But all of mine will be.

MARY HALTER PETERSEN
Joseph, Utah

When I was pregnant for the first time I was not yet vegetarian, and ate a typical American diet full of meat and animal products. My blood pressure during that pregnancy was on the very high end of what was considered normal. I was under no particular additional stress and I've come to associate that borderline hypertension with my high meat diet.

By the time I conceived my second child I'd been a non-meat-eating vegetarian for seven months. Thinking I had to eat animal protein to get enough protein, I still ate quite a lot of dairy products and eggs. I experienced none of the high blood pressure during that pregnancy. My baby was quite large at birth—8 pounds, 11 ounces—and I was quite uncomfortable those last weeks of pregnancy. She also had quite a lot of mucus at birth which required a lot of suctioning to clear.

Since we were planning a do-it-yourself home birth with our third child I wanted to be as careful as I could be with my/our health. I had read a book by a Utah midwife that said she notices more mucus and breathing problems in babies whose mothers had eaten dairy products during their pregnancy, so I decided to delete most of them from my diet. I had been decreasing my intake of dairy products anyway so it wasn't that big a transition.

I'd read enough about the personal, cultural and planetary health problems associated with eating animal products to be convinced to focus on an essentially vegan diet. I especially benefited from John Robbins's *Diet for a New America*, Dr. Michael Klaper's books—*Pregnancy, Children and the Vegan Diet* and *Vegan Nutrition: Pure and Simple*—and *Transition to Vegetarianism* by Rudolph Ballentine.

I'd also heard of someone conducting research on baby size and traditional diets, i.e., diets consisting of mainly grains and vegetables. The researcher wanted to show that babies *in utero* grow just as healthy, but not as large when the mother eats a grain-based diet, making birth easier for both mother and baby. Without hearing more, it made sense to me. Healthy babies have been born for centuries all over the world in cultures where the consumption of animal products, meat, dairy or eggs, is almost non-existent. And there never seem to be stories in meat-eating cultures like the ones from non-meat-eating cultures of women stepping off to the side during the course of their day, birthing their babies and returning to their work. Birth stories indicative of easier labors and births are most often associated with diet, as well as with the level of physical fitness.

During my third pregnancy, I didn't worry about protein combinations within one meal since becoming aware of the latest research that shows our bodies do indeed have their own wisdom and are quite capable of making complete proteins from the components of several meals. During the first few months of pregnancy and for several weeks postpartum I did crave eggs, so I ate those along with my otherwise grain- and vegetable-based diet. The only dairy I ate was a very occasional yogurt, which usually make me feel kind of foggy, so I eventually stopped eating even that. I felt healthy and strong throughout the pregnancy and feel that my diet supplied all the nutrients I and my baby needed.

Occasionally, I did take various vitamin and mineral supplements, I guess as a kind of insurance that I was getting what I needed, especially during the first four months, when nausea sometimes prevented me from eating as well as I might have. I never took any supplement on a daily basis because I didn't want my body to rely on artificial sources of nutrition. I just continued to find a variety of vegetable and grain sources of the vitamins and minerals I felt I needed most.

I didn't visit any doctors or midwives during my pregnancy as I had with my first two. I didn't believe that their external measurements could tell me that I was healthy more than my own responsibility and awareness could. I had found in my first two pregnancies that visiting a doctor had prevented me from believing in my own body's wisdom by putting the focus on their equipment and what it said about my body, instead of assisting me in listening to my own state of health that I experienced by living it. And in so many ways I felt so much better, more tuned in to my own needs, my baby's needs, more focused on truest responsibility and fullest health.

My daughter was born after a rather easy labor. She had just a tiny bit of mucus in her mouth. She was healthy, well and beautiful. She weighed 7 pounds and had beautiful color and healthy, glowing skin. I kept marveling at the smoothness and clarity of her skin. My first two babies' skin had been much more mottled and uneven in color and appearance.

My daughter is almost one year old now and weighs almost 20 pounds. We've continued a diet almost totally free of all animal products, essentially living on a diet of varied grains, dried beans, vegetables and some fruits. I regained my pre-pregnancy size within three to four months of birth and have maintained an abundant milk supply throughout this first year. I feel healthier than I ever did and my baby is bright and happy, learning to walk and already saying 15 to 20 words, new ones every day.

My period has yet to return, with breast-feeding and perhaps diet also influencing a welcome respite from fertility. My period returned by eight months even though I was totally breast-feeding my first two children, so the only other difference aside from my age and number of children is in my diet.

I feel that my vegetarian diet gave my daughter the best possible start in life, free from the health problems associated with animal foods and with a physical clarity that influences a mental, emotional and spiritual clarity as well.

I felt better during this last pregnancy than I did with either of my previous pregnancies and I feel my diet supplied my baby and me with all the nutrients we both needed for optimal health and growth. I was never worried about not getting enough, and I was relieved of the worry of giving my baby all the toxins that are present in animal products to such a concentrated degree. I ate healthy, read a lot, exercised and believed in our health, and I felt it!

LAURA PETSCHING
Oxford, Massachusetts

My first child, Seth, was born by caesarean on May 26, 1989. I had always been a meat-eater and did not think of changing my diet when pregnant. While I was pregnant, I worked as a nurse three nights a week. I was very tired during my first trimester, but never suffered any nausea or vomiting.

Seth began eating solid food at five-and-a-half months (fruits, vegetables, and grains). When Seth was seven months old, I became a vegetarian for health and environmental reasons. Seth has never eaten meat. He is of average height and very slim. My husband and I are both slim so this is not worrisome.

When I became pregnant with Anna, I had been vegetarian for about 15 months. All the popular literature warned that vegetarians cannot get enough protein when pregnant. I had read about studies conducted by Dr. Tom Brewer which linked eclampsia to inadequate protein intake. To reassure myself that the protein in my diet was adequate, I kept a food diary for one week and had it evaluated by a dietitian. She assured me that I was getting plenty of protein and vitamins.

During my second pregnancy, I did not work outside the home. Again, I was very tired during the first trimester. I did suffer some nausea with this pregnancy, but I attribute that to fatigue as Seth was still not sleeping through the night and did not wean until I was about four-and-a-half months pregnant. Anna was born at home on January 5, 1992. She weighed 9 pounds and was 21 inches long—2 pounds heavier than her brother had been and 1 inch longer. Obviously, vegetarian women do not have tinier or sicker babies than meat-eating women.

Becoming a vegetarian did not affect my milk supply. While nursing both children I have had a plentiful supply and have been able to pump milk to store for emergencies and to donate to a milk bank.

We are lacto-ovo vegetarians, eating dairy products and baking with eggs. Neither of my children has ever been on antibiotics or been hospitalized. Overall, I would say that our diet keeps us very healthy.

KIM PICKETT-DEPAOLIS
Hammond, Louisiana

During my first pregnancy four years ago, I still ate seafood so I had no real concerns about protein or iron intake. But right after Joshua was born, we stopped eating seafood and became committed vegetarians. When I became pregnant again, I was sure that a vegetarian diet was very healthy for myself and my baby. For my husband Rory, Josh and me, vegetarianism had become a deeply rooted part of our lives.

Because we were planning a home birth, that issue overshadowed the vegetarian pregnancy as far as our families were concerned. But we were lucky to receive loving support for our decisions. The only resistance I met was from the nutritionist at the WIC (Women, Infants and Children) program. Her concern was that I was pregnant and still nursing Josh; she felt I wouldn't get the proper nutrients to nourish my baby. My iron count was determined to be low so she suggested that I eat some meat or wean Josh.

I knew she meant well, but neither of her solutions were acceptable to me. A nurse practitioner suggested that I take iron supplements. I followed her advice and three days later developed a kidney infection.

At the same time, I happened to be reading Susun Weed's *Wise Woman's Herbal for the Childbearing Years*. In it, she said that iron supplements can cause kidney infections because they are difficult for the kidneys to process and the iron is not absorbed well anyway. She offered a recipe for an iron tonic made from yellow dock root. I took one to two tablespoons a day and my iron count soared! Maybe low iron levels are common for vegetarians during pregnancy, but iron supplements or consuming meat would, I feel, hurt more than help.

With my first pregnancy, I was a protein fanatic. But with pregnancy number two I wasn't as conscientious. On average I got 60 to 70 grams of protein a day and I felt confident that I was getting a healthy amount. But sometimes I would crave meat. And the cravings were for McDonald's-type food, of all things! These cravings occurred only a few times over the course of my last two trimesters. I knew my body was telling me I needed more protein at those particular times, but peanut butter, beans, soy products, even cheese would not satisfy me. If I ate eggs, which we rarely did, the craving was subdued. But my belief is that no animal products are necessary for a healthy pregnancy so I do wonder about the source of that craving.

My pregnancy ended with a magnificent birth! Caleb weighed 9 pounds, 4 ounces and, like his brother Josh, has been very healthy. Our family is heading down a vegan path—we're trying! At three-and-a-half years, Josh is still nursing and Caleb at nine months is a very hearty nurser. I have no doubts that a vegetarian diet can provide nutritionally for a healthy start to a baby's life.

JULIE A. PRYCHITKO
Oswego, New York

I was confident and comfortable with my diet, having been a vegetarian for two years before becoming pregnant. I thought I had heard all the questions about vegetarianism. But as my expanding belly announced my pregnancy to the world, women everywhere felt it was their duty to examine my eating habits.

My first prenatal visit was with a nurse-midwife during my fifth week of pregnancy. She surprised my husband Andre when she claimed to be a vegetarian who eats chicken and fish. She tried to convince me of the value of eating fish during my pregnancy, which disturbed me because of the current research I had heard: infants whose mothers ate fish from the Great Lakes region (where we live) during pregnancy were found to have significantly high amounts of birth defects. I did not eat any fish while I was pregnant, because I never liked it, even before choosing to become a vegetarian.

I took about 150 of the prenatal vitamins that were so strongly recommended to me by our midwife until my system became so clogged that I couldn't stand it any more. I also tried taking the Slow Fe iron tablets suggested to me after a blood test in my 30th week of pregnancy revealed that I had anemia; after two tablets daily for a couple of weeks, my body rejected them also. So I went back to my normal eating pattern.

During my 23rd week of pregnancy, my husband and I attended a friend's baptism. I was stuffed with salads, vegetables, lasagna, eggplant Parmesan, and cake by the end of the baptismal party, when Aunt Mary introduced herself to me. She said something like, "Hi, I'm Aunt Mary. It was nice meeting you." We had just met that moment. "Give me a hug. So, you're a vegetarian . . . what do you eat?"

As I pointed out the many delicious Italian entrees I had just eaten, I noticed that all eyes were on me. Several of the elderly women had quite a discussion about my apparently radical eating choices during pregnancy. But they all wished me good luck as they left the party.

My husband and I started childbirth education classes during my 31st week of pregnancy. I knew they would seem endless when I was told, at our first session, to drink four glasses of milk a day and to eat red meat at least three times a week. When we asked [the group leader] what a pregnant vegetarian should eat, she replied, "I don't know. I'm not an expert in nutrition." At least she was honest.

I trusted my instincts for healthy eating during my pregnancy. After four long months of "evening sickness," I ate constantly. I ate bushels of fruit, especially melons and bananas. I loved carrots, cucumbers and peppers, while lettuce turned my stomach. I ate many vegetable omelettes and egg salad sandwiches, because I craved eggs more than usual. I enjoyed steamed vegetables on a bed of brown rice. My favorite bedtime snack was cereal topped with sliced bananas and soy milk. I loved blueberry pancakes and apple spice muffins.

I ate just about everything in sight, so I tried to keep junk food out of the house. However, I did give in to chocolate, donuts and coffee more often than I care to admit. I drank continually—gallons of distilled water and fresh citrus juice. If I become pregnant again, I will add plenty (four to six glasses a day) of fresh vegetable juices to my daily diet.

I strongly advise pregnant women to trust their instincts, even when pressure from well-meaning friends, relatives or childbirth instructors suggests otherwise, when it comes to eating. You know your body better than anyone else.

SAMANTHA RAFFERTY
Brooklyn, New York

I am a lacto-ovo vegetarian mother. When I became pregnant three years ago (with triplets!), I met with resistance and ignorance from the medical community, not to mention most of my family.

My doctor told me that if I "insisted" on being a vegetarian, I had to eat four eggs a day. It is truly amazing how many doctors know next to nothing about nutrition!

I have been a vegetarian for five years but never ate well because I did it due to personal convictions about eating meat rather than for health reasons. Trying to find a way to have a healthy pregnancy was almost impossible. But both your books (*Vegetarian Baby* and *Vegetarian Children*) and Rose Eliot's book, *The Vegetarian Mother and Baby Book*, got me through it.

When I was 11½ weeks pregnant, I miscarried the fraternal baby (I now have identical twin boys). My doctor blamed me. He told me I was at fault because I "refused to do the right thing and eat fish and meat."

I continued through my pregnancy as a vegetarian. I gave birth 10 weeks early which was, of course, blamed on my diet. But my boys were both over 4 pounds at birth, whereas most children born at 30 weeks' gestation are usually only

3 pounds. Believe me, when they are that small, a single pound makes a world of difference.

I have since found a very supportive pediatrician who calls my sons the "Tofu Twins." I am convinced that my children are alive and healthy today because I continued my vegetarian diet throughout pregnancy and because they too are vegetarians now.

NANCY RANKIN
Seattle, Washington

I had been a macrobiotic cooking teacher six years prior to motherhood, and made a lot of decisions about how I thought I was going to eat during pregnancy. It was my first lesson in what now has been a perpetual ritual of "letting go."

I was exactly six weeks into my pregnancy when all my preconceived ideas went out the window. I became extremely nauseous, and could no more have conceived of eating brown rice and miso soup, than stood in my kitchen to prepare it. For the first half of my pregnancy, I subsisted on endless bowls of cereal, soy milk and fruit. This was not the diet I had imagined I would consume to nourish my baby. I didn't fit my own model for a well-nourished pregnancy. My body had ideas of its own. I began to listen and trust.

Gradually, my tastes widened and I began to handle more substantial fare. Whole grains, beans, land and sea vegetables, nuts and seeds once again graced my plate with increasing proportion. As I had abstained from dairy for many years, I was surprised one day to find myself staring at the yogurt section in the co-op. I weighed the chatter in my head with my body's process to be attracted to foods that corresponded to my changing nutritional needs. I listened to my body. The yogurt tasted and felt appropriate. I redefined my macrobiotic label to reflect the art of making balance.

SUSANNA ROSENBAUM
Montreal, Canada

I am 32 years old and the mother of four boys, all born within a six-year period. I followed a vegetarian diet throughout all four pregnancies. When I decided to have a fourth child, my diet was the most "radical" or "restrictive" that it had ever been. I saw no need to change once I became pregnant. I just had to listen to my body and eat a wide variety of foods in sufficient quantities.

When I was pregnant for the first time, nearly seven years ago, I forced myself to eat two eggs and drink a litre of milk every day. From the reading that I had done, and from the advice of my friends and family, I felt that this was the only way to guarantee an adequate protein and calcium intake during pregnancy while following a vegetarian diet. I gained 40 pounds and I looked as if I were carrying a basketball under my shirt by the time nine months had gone by. My baby weighed about 9 pounds at birth.

I became pregnant for the second time less than a year after the birth of my first son. That pregnancy was very different. I still tried to force myself to eat eggs and milk but I had very little appetite and ate a lot of junk food, if that was what I felt like having at any given moment. I gained 27 pounds and my baby was a healthy 7½ pounds.

When I was pregnant almost a year-and-a-half later, I was being cared for by a midwife as well as being followed by a doctor. The midwife told me that if I didn't feel like drinking milk, I didn't have to. There are many sources of calcium and she saw no reason to think that my diet was deficient in protein or any other essential nutrients. I also nursed my toddler throughout my third pregnancy. I gained 43 pounds and, 17 days past my due date, I gave birth to an 8-pound, 3-ounce boy at home. As the months went by, it became clear that my third son was sensitive to many foods in my diet. I eventually stopped drinking milk altogether and greatly reduced the dairy products I was eating.

When I decided to have a fourth child, I was feeling great on a fairly low-fat, almost vegan diet. I did not change my diet once I became pregnant. I was nursing a toddler once again, but not very much, and he did in fact wean during my pregnancy. I was again being cared for by a midwife as well as a doctor. However, I was extremely busy and active during my pregnancy and had a great deal of trouble gaining any weight at all. I did not gain an ounce until I was already five months pregnant. I attempted to add more fat and dairy products to my diet, but I could not tolerate them and had trouble with indigestion and constipation. I was not worried about my health nor was my midwife. My doctor was less sure. My belly was smaller than it should have been considering how far along I should have been. I was not gaining much weight and my blood tests showed a certain amount of anemia. This was the same doctor who had followed me through my three previous pregnancies.

For the first time I was being pressured by my doctor, my friends and my family (with the exception of my husband) about my overall health and of course about my "restricted vegetarian diet." One visit to my parents' house during my pregnancy was extremely stressful. Everyone was watching every bite that I took; the result, of course, was that I felt even less like eating and had more indigestion!

The midwife felt that my baby was healthy and he was very active. My doctor, however, insisted that I get an ultrasound at 37 weeks, which confirmed that the baby and placenta were both fine, although the baby was only average in size. I took an herbal iron supplement and additional iron because of the anemia shown by my blood tests, but I refused to eat liver, as one friend suggested, or to drink milk, which practically everyone seemed to think would be some kind of magic health tonic.

In the end, I gained only 20 pounds. Except for several colds that I caught from my children and some varicose veins from being on my feet so much, I felt great throughout my pregnancy. I was very tired, but I don't think it was because of my diet. My baby was born ten days past my due date, again at home. He was small, 6 pounds, 9 ounces, and in perfect health. The placenta was also quite healthy. My midwife felt that the baby was smaller than my others *not* because he hadn't been adequately nourished *in utero*, but because he had been so active that he never really put on any fat.

Sym Robin is now four months old: a big and fat baby who weighs about 18 pounds. I have breast-fed all of my children while following a vegetarian diet. The older three were all 20 pounds by six months of age and I have always had problems with an over-supply of milk. My experience over the last seven years has shown me that it is perfectly possible to be a vegetarian, have healthy pregnancies and then breast-feed without any problems, only very healthy children.

VALERIE SCHULTZ
Tehachapi, California

It was a family affair: my husband Randy, our three daughters and I all became vegetarians together. We decided to try life without meat for one month in February of 1989. We have not eaten any meat since.

Our two older daughters, Morgan and Zoe, were six and four at the time. They were relieved not to be eating creatures with whom they felt a spiritual kinship and whose taste they abhorred anyway. Our youngest, Raven, was six months old and still breast-feeding exclusively; the only meat that ever crossed her lips was through my breast milk, prior to [our lifestyle change]. Randy and I became vegans (he did before I did). The children continued to eat eggs and dairy products. We were all lean and healthy and free of guilt.

We decided in the cold of winter to have one more baby, and conceived our fourth daughter in January 1991. It was the night the ground war began in the Persian Gulf and I remember thinking that couples all over the country might be responding to the news as we were, by making extra love, giving this time more than its share of conceptions.

As I had done when we first became vegetarians, I read everything I could find on the subject of vegetarian and vegan pregnancy: magazines, books, interviews, cookbooks, medical journals. As with any controversial subject, contradictions abounded, but what I read largely reassured me that this vegetarian pregnancy would be a healthy one.

I did not tell my doctor that I had become a vegetarian since my last pregnancy, because I didn't want to have to defend myself (I felt like a coward, though). I simply answered "yes" when he asked if I was eating well. After three pregnancies, he was used to me: I was a strange but model patient. I refused all prenatal testing and as many birth interventions as possible, nursed my kids for a long time and used only the Billings Ovulation Method of natural birth control. I was the medical equivalent of a cheap date.

During my first trimester, what I thought was morning sickness turned out to be a lengthy bout of stomach flu. After a few weeks of debilitating illness, I wildly craved yogurt. At the same time, I read that infants of nursing vegan mothers are the highest risk group for B_{12} deficiency. Even though my head knew a vegan pregnancy was perfectly viable, my nerves gave in to my doubts. That day I returned to lacto-ovo vegetarian status, eating yogurt at least once a day for the rest of my pregnancy.

Another dietary change during that pregnancy involved beans. I had embraced the poetry in the image of the pot of beans soaking in my kitchen: sorting and soaking different varieties of beans had become an almost daily family ritual. But during the first three months of this pregnancy, I could barely stand the thought of beans. One night I cooked up a batch of Portuguese beans—a family favorite—and burst into tears at the sight of them steaming in my bowl. A long while passed before I ate beans again. And even then I started small—with lentils.

Otherwise, my pregnancy proceeded smoothly. I worried about protein intake and took an iron supplement—both needlessly. By my last month I experienced heartburn, so I rarely ate a whole meal. Drinking milk relieved this. Then in the last few weeks, my fingers retained water and often felt numb. Finally, I had to have my wedding ring cut off, which was pretty upsetting. But I think what upset me more than these problems was my reaction to them: my own brain discourteously kept blaming my vegetarian diet. I didn't need friends or relatives or parents scaring me; I was doing it to myself. Fortunately, Randy remained supportive of my diet and pointed this out: I had never blamed problems in previous pregnancies on the fact that I ate meat and yet look at all the problems meat causes!

Mariah Earth arrived six days late, weighing 7 pounds, 15 ounces, only 4 ounces less than her lightest sibling. My labor this time was hard, but efficient, which I attribute to the daily cup of raspberry leaf tea I drank throughout pregnancy. The moment she was placed on my chest, she lifted her head right up and gazed at me! Such strength, I thought. Must be because she's a vegetarian. And she began to nurse, my first and only meat-free baby from Day One. Mariah is now six months old and has yet to be ill. She has had no colic, no jaundice, no ear infections or allergies. She is smart and loving, peaceful and happy, active and rosy. Draw your own conclusions!

LYNN I. SEMEGA
Olympia, Washington

At age 38, I felt in the prime of my life. My weight was low and stable, my body strong, my complexion clear. I had been a vegetarian since 1975, when I had given up meat and fish for both moral and health reasons. The diet had become second nature and it seemed as though I'd never eaten meat. I consumed some dairy products, mostly raw milk and humane dairy farm products, and I ate eggs once a week for breakfast.

I was in my 17th year teaching elementary school in inner-city Cleveland, Ohio. When friends called to arrange a 100-mile bike ride, I never hesitated. I'd smile to myself as we sped by male riders. In short, I was a healthy, single vegetarian woman, with a lifelong desire to be a mother in the back of my mind.

Many of my friends who were approaching 40 were having fertility problems. Some had been trying for years to conceive. I had one unprotected night with my boyfriend and ended up pregnant. I believe that my good health via a vegetarian diet kept my body young and able to conceive easily. Because it was totally unplanned, David and I were frantic, but thrilled.

My first reaction was to meet with an obstetrician; I had a lot of questions and concerns about my age and possible complications. I was enrolled in a group program through my employer and assigned to an Indian physician. He acknowledged that many women in his country were vegetarian throughout their pregnancies, but recommended that I supplement my diet with fish for the coming nine months. I did not agree and so he wanted me to add a multiple vitamin, followed by an iron supplement, to my diet. I told him I was sure I could get all the nutrients I needed from whole foods, but he insisted on the supplements.

My first two months went smoothly. I hardly knew I was pregnant. I never experienced a moment of morning sickness. I felt wonderful and continued to hike with friends. However, near the end of the second month, I started to bleed. It was copious enough for me to rush to my doctor's office. He was worried and decided I needed total bed rest, in consideration of my age.

I didn't feel old, but I went along with his suggestion because I was deathly afraid of losing my chance to have the baby. He instructed me to stay off my feet as much as possible, not to drive my car, and of course, not to work for at least four weeks. I filed for sick leave and stayed home, coming back for the last two days of school only. Mostly, I stayed in bed with my feet propped up higher than my stomach, as recommended. My diet remained exemplary, with grains, vegetables and fresh fruits. I tried to drink plenty of water, too. The four weeks crawled by.

At the beginning of my second trimester, ultrasound revealed placenta previa. No more blood appeared, but the doctor told me that this condition meant a caesarean section at term. I felt very discouraged.

My mother urged me every day to "drink more milk—gallons of it." I had never really enjoyed milk, but I did add at least a cup of yogurt to my diet, in case my mother knew best.

When I was four months pregnant, David and I moved to Washington state in a pick-up truck with a U-haul, automobile and small trailer, a Malamute dog and four cats. The ride took us through extremes of temperature. I relied on fresh fruit stands to get me through. I craved peaches, plums and all kinds of berries. In spite of having to sleep in the front seat of a truck, I fared quite well.

My third trimester was exhilarating. The placenta previa resolved itself as the fetus grew larger. I was tired and slower, but I felt great. My weight started to skyrocket as I developed an intense craving for ice cream, chocolate, and other sugar-laden treats. I knew it wasn't the best thing, but I felt like I deserved the treats.

My new obstetrician was a woman. She was very comfortable with my vegetarianism, but in the eighth month, my iron level dropped below the recommended levels. She prescribed iron supplements, which I took until delivery. I went to a health food store and was able to find a suitable vegetable-based supplement instead of the liver-based iron she had prescribed.

Three weeks before my son, Flint, was born, David and I got married in our backyard. He is a staunch vegetarian, too, and he was with me all the way on matters of diet. In matters of the heart, he came through with a lifetime commitment just before the big moment! We feasted on freshly squeezed carrot juice and a triple chocolate torte that day.

Even though I was eating mass quantities of everything, I maintained a good balance of healthy foods each day. I wanted this baby to come out healthy and strong.

The birth was not smooth. After 22 hours of intense labor, the doctor decided a caesarean was necessary. I went home with my 8-pound, 6-ounce, 22-inch son five days later. He came out perfect, with an Apgar score of 9 and looking great! (Note: for caesarean births, a 9 score is considered excellent.)

My son is now 3½ years old. I nursed him for two-and-a-half years, keeping up a super diet of fresh, whole foods. I still ate dairy and eggs once a week, but I cut out the sweets. My son has never tasted flesh foods and is extremely healthy. He is now 43 inches tall and weighs 40 pounds, measuring up in size to children two years older.

I have friends nearby who are also raising veggie children, and my parents have retired near us. They support my decision to raise Flint as a vegetarian. Life is good!

LINDA TAGLIAFERRO
Little Neck, New York

At 4'11" and 90 pounds, I was not the type of person you would expect to run into at an all-you-can-eat buffet. Yet when I became pregnant at the age of 31, I could suddenly pack it away like Hulk Hogan.

For the first and only time in my life, I realized what it meant to be hungry. I decided early in my pregnancy that there would be no hard and fast rules as to what I would or would not eat, as long as it was healthy food. I would let my body do the choosing. I gave in to cravings for specific fruits, occasional potato binges, and even a very un-vegetarian desire for bay scallops in particular (sea scallops wouldn't do). Had I wanted to eat meat, I would have, but I have never found meat more repulsive than in those nine months. The result of following my instincts was that I remained healthy and physically active, and my pregnancy culminated in a wonderful home birth.

I became an "official" vegetarian when I was 11, although my mother affirms that I hated meat even as a three-year-old. I still ate fish, eggs and dairy until my late 20s, when I eliminated them from my diet. However, I didn't escape the lure of sour cream and goat cheese.

One thing that was noteworthy about my pregnancy was that I was on "automatic pilot" nutritionally. I ate rich soups of avocado and kombu, a mineral-rich sea vegetable, until my hair got even thicker, longer and healthier-looking than my pre-pregnancy tresses.

I reveled in high-nutrition snacks like sunflower seeds and fruits. With the exception of an occasional first-trimester bout of queasiness, I continued to be physically active. I awoke with morning sickness one day into my second month, but managed to perform in a Balinese dance recital that evening and felt great! I joked that my son was such an active toddler because I danced so much during my pregnancy.

I had a strong craving for milk. Those who avoid dairy will disagree with my choice to imbibe a full quart a day but, at that time, I could still buy drug-free raw milk.

At the beginning of my pregnancy I followed the advice of an acquaintance who was the mother of three children. She recommended a tasty German tonic called Floradix, which has a fabulous fruit flavor and is high in easy-to-assimilate iron. Around my eighth month, I also started taking wheat grass tablets on the advice of another vegetarian mother who had been anemic, but cured the problem with them.

I also had the advice of a wonderful nurse-midwife, since I gave birth to my son, Eric, at home. She set very high standards for the health of the women whose babies she agreed to deliver and so I had frequent blood tests to check my hematocrit. Finally, after taking Floradix and wheat grass tablets, I joyfully heard these words, "Linda, what are you taking? I want to tell all my other clients! Your hematocrit is so good that I'm going to stop doing blood tests." Balm to my sore fingertips!

Another supplement I took frequently was raspberry leaf tea, which all the herbal books described as *the* supplement for pregnant moms. It's so pleasant, if not bland, and contained so many vitamins and nutrients that I felt no need to take a vitamin supplement. In general, I feel that whole foods and herbs are better absorbed than pills.

The home birth was beautiful and peaceful. It was more like having my husband and a friend around than a medical experience. By the time Eric was 2, I went down to 5 pounds under my pre-pregnancy weight. I attribute this to breast-feeding (I think everything I ate went through me right into Eric) and running around after a super-healthy toddler.

That was years ago. Eric is now a healthy vegetarian child and I don't have to run after him as much. Things have calmed down so much that I even tip the scale at 103 pounds—a record for me.

If I was going to do it again, I wouldn't change a thing. My advice: stick to healthy foods, and just trust your instincts.

LONNA WILKINSON
Washington, D.C.

I have been a vegetarian for over 20 years, through two pregnancies, the second one with twins. The elimination of meat in my diet was a gradual and natural evolution, dictated largely by the positive response of my body, and it never felt like a deprivation. Though I limit the amount, I eat eggs and dairy products. I occasionally eat fish, especially if I am at a restaurant with few other vegetarian options. My husband of 15 years is not a vegetarian and sometimes orders meat in sandwiches and at restaurants. But we do not cook meat at home and we are both comfortable with this arrangement.

Pregnancy was a very interesting experience, particularly regarding my relationship to food. Eating became a clear function of my body's emphatic and fairly specific demands, which overrode any previous habitual or more conscious choices. During the first trimester especially, I noticed several changes in my food desires. I soon found I was eating eggs and dairy in greater amounts than before. This seemed to be the simplest and most satisfying way to meet my body's demands for protein. Strangely, foods that I normally avoided, and considered to be greasy, salty or processed, suddenly caught my eye. At work, I was amazed to find myself drooling over the university cafeteria food and to find that pizza, Fritos and other vending machine snacks seemed irresistible. My only explanation is that I was hungry all the time, and since these foods were readily available, they took on a new appeal. I did carry healthy snacks with me, but if

I found myself salivating over the institutional spaghetti, lasagna, pizza or daily special, I was happy to indulge.

I actually got quite a kick out of these odd food requests from my body and I was happy to let my appetite and tastes run further afield than they had in many years. Pregnancy seemed like a particularly appropriate time to let my body guide the way, and I was happy let go of some of the more mentally controlled eating habits I usually rely upon. It was interesting to notice also, that once pregnancy was over, these foods did not retain their appeal nor did I have to struggle to get my eating back on track.

Also during the first trimester, my interest in salt was at an all-time high, but I did not desire sweets or sugar at all. In fact, sweets did not have any appeal whatsoever until the last few months of pregnancy. The only aversion I ever developed was for Mexican food, which was surprising because it is usually standard fare in our house.

During the second trimester, when the nausea and intense hunger had subsided, I started wanting foods that I associated with childhood. I rediscovered applesauce, graham crackers, cottage cheese, oatmeal and a special brunch pancake my mother used to make—all foods I had not eaten for many years. I did, however, draw the line at a desire for liverwurst and mustard sandwiches. But I considered that this craving might indicate a need for iron and I was careful to increase my intake of that nutrient through other foods.

Family members who had, over time, come to accept and even partially adopt my eating habits were suddenly doubtful once again about the nutritional soundness of my diet. Fears of toxemia, anemia, premature birth and concern for brain development were gently broached in long distance phone calls. Although I certainly had anxieties during my pregnancy, I was absolutely comfortable with my diet and able to fend off these well-intentioned reproaches with relative equanimity.

My pregnancy continued normally. I gained 40 pounds and gave birth to a beautiful 8-pound, 2-ounce baby girl. My daughter, Berkeley, is now three-and-a-half and a robust, healthy vegetarian.

A week before my 40th birthday I went in for a routine sonogram before having CVS genetic testing. I was 11 weeks into my second pregnancy and once again experiencing a constant low-level nausea. Nothing I tried, including saltines, special teas, acupressure bands on my wrists, or eating many small meals, seemed to provide any relief. I was also, as had been true with my first pregnancy, craving salt and eating odd junk food items that I usually never touch. Everything seemed normal and then the technician told me I was having twins.

My pregnancy was then categorized as high risk due to the twins, my age and a previous caesarean section. My doctor, who was fairly traditional in his training and approach, saw no problem with my vegetarian diet, especially since I was eating eggs and dairy. He prescribed prenatal vitamins and sent me on my way. I was relieved that I was not going to be asked to re-evaluate my diet; my experience with my first baby gave me confidence that my vegetarian diet was a great plus in having a healthy pregnancy.

My twin pregnancy seemed even easier than my first, except that towards the end I was uncomfortable because my belly was so enormous. The food cravings were similar, but they didn't seem as extreme, perhaps because it was the second time around and perhaps because we were busy moving. With one highly energetic child already, there was less time to attend to my body's cravings.

In my reading on twin pregnancies, some schools of thought emphasized significant weight gain (50 to 80 pounds) as being a key factor in having a full-term pregnancy and avoiding low birth weights. My intuition told me to eat healthfully and whatever amount was comfortable, but not to eat just to gain weight, hungry or not. I don't think I ate more than during my first pregnancy, although the notion of "eating for three" was sometimes tempting. I gained 45 pounds and my pregnancy was full term. I gave birth to twin boys, Graham who weighed 7 pounds, and Geoffrey who weighed 7½ pounds—high birth weights for twins. At birth they were healthy, happy, active and alert boys, and so they are now at seven months—excellent examples of healthy vegetarian babies born from a vegetarian pregnancy.

My decision to be a vegetarian was an intuitive one, not based on any particular philosophy, and lacking in detailed expertise, although I did spend several years initially learning to reorient my cooking. I have never been comfortable making my diet the focus of a lot of attention or trouble, and I have never proselytized for vegetarianism. However, over time I have come to realize what a subtle, but significant and positive effect my choice has had on my health and my life, and the lives of those around me. Vegetarianism is my own quiet and personal protest against the status quo and against a world order based on hierarchy, whether it be people over animals, men over women, or race over race. I encourage other women in their choices to have vegetarian pregnancies and raise vegetarian children, and affirm that choice with my own experience.

CAROLINE ZIOGAS
Springfield, Illinois

At age 14, I was exposed to the idea of a vegetarian diet, but still ate meat. By age 16, I had become a vegetarian. A few months after I turned 17, I became pregnant. I was attending college and working part-time. Naturally, I was fatigued, but very excited.

When my doctor found out I was a vegetarian, she had me visit a dietitian. The dietitian turned out to be most helpful and concerned. She gave me a reprint of an article called "Vegetarian Nutrition." It was through her that I learned about complete proteins. She recommended the books *Laurel's Kitchen* and *Diet for a Small Planet*.

The dietitian suggested I log what I ate day to day, so that she and my doctor could check it. I learned to be careful about proteins. When I asked the dietitian what was most important to pay attention to, she said calcium and protein, and recommended I try to consume 100 grams of protein a day. I never felt any criticism from either her or my doctor as they gave me the information I needed. My husband also decided to become a vegetarian during this time, so he was supportive also.

I wanted what was best for my baby and felt that a vegetarian diet would be of most benefit. I was careful to avoid caffeine, although I did eat chocolate at times. I really craved oranges, especially during my third trimester. For snacks, I enjoyed crackers and cheese. I never was a milk fan, but I forced myself to drink it because I felt it was better for my baby. I enjoyed fruit juices and smoothies, to which I added wheat germ, yogurt, fruit, powdered milk, ice cream and, at times, juice. My husband made homemade lemonade. I loved having a salad with everything in it for a meal.

There were times I felt nauseated, particularly after dinner and in the evenings. My weight gain was about 50 pounds but my doctor did not give me a hard time about it. I was never anemic.

Near my due date, I developed pre-eclampsia. I had edema and my blood pressure was high. My doctor ordered 48 hours of bed rest and urged me to drink plenty of liquids along with a good diet. I did what she said, only getting up to use the bathroom. This helped and, thereafter, I gave myself regular periods of rest, propping my feet up.

I had no medication during labor and on July 4th at 5:52 A.M., my son, Benjamin Lee Ziogas, was born. He was 8 pounds, 4 ounces and 21½ inches long. I nursed him in the recovery room. He was given extra iron for a while, because his umbilical cord was cut before he was born, so he didn't get the extra iron-rich blood. He grew wonderfully, in the 50th to 90th percentiles for weight and length.

In 1987, I became pregnant again. I really looked forward to this pregnancy also. I had a different doctor this time. I found out she was a vegetarian and shared my concerns with her as to whether a vegetarian diet would be enough for a second pregnancy. My nutrition fears caused me to eat part of a tuna sandwich. Her answer was, "Why should it be different now, as long as you have a good diet during pregnancy?" which reassured me. I realized my fears were unfounded and continued with my normal vegetarian diet. When my iron level was tested, my doctor said it was excellent.

The doctor also told me about current research which indicates that you don't have to eat complete proteins at each meal as long as you do so by the end of the day. This was very interesting and made it much easier to eat complete proteins every day.

There was a Bradley childbirth instructor in town and we decided to take classes. The diet called for 100 grams of protein a day. When I mentioned being a vegetarian to the instructor, she did not seem concerned. When I was in my last trimester, however, she suggested eating liver once a week. I told her I wouldn't be eating liver because I did not eat meat. She didn't push the issue and went on to other subjects. When we charted our diet for a week, my protein intake was fine.

The doctor became concerned about my weight gain during the third trimester, because it was disappointing compared to earlier gains in my pregnancy weight. I continued to eat what I wanted, craving oranges off and on. I ate two eggs a day, which was recommended by the Bradley method. My weight gain by the end turned out to be about 45 pounds. When Hannah Mary was born, she weighed 7 pounds, 6 ounces and her length was 20 inches, with an Apgar score of 9 to 10.

When Hannah was nine months old, I became pregnant with my third child. I had nausea but it ended at 11½ weeks. [At term,] my weight gain was 26 pounds, my hematocrit was 13, and Ruth Cora weighed 8 pounds, 4 ounces and was 20½ inches long.

When Ruth was a year old, I became pregnant again. I was still nursing her. It was important for me to eat six or more times a day. My hunger was intense and my energy level would drop off if I did not snack often. I took prenatal vitamins occasionally, but a lot was going on so I sometimes forgot. My iron level was still good and I gained about 25 pounds. Isabel Rebekah weighed 8 pounds at birth and was 20¾ inches long.

I nursed through two of my pregnancies and I had three daughters close in age. All my children are growing and healthy. The nourishment from my lacto-ovo vegetarian diet continues to be adequate, if not superior, even through these demanding times.

Chapter Three

Common Concerns

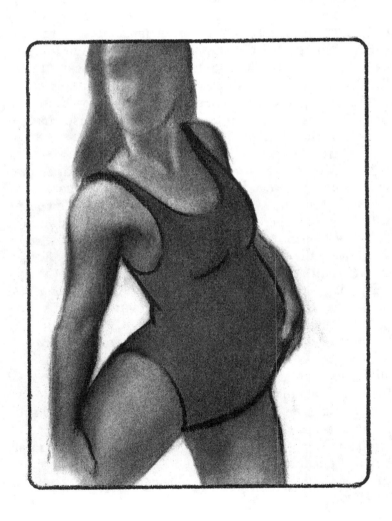

No matter where they live in the world, no matter how much they have learned about nutrition, pregnant women think about many of the same things. As a woman's body changes, she is likely to have concerns about the nausea of early pregnancy, weight gain, her energy level and unusual food cravings. But, depending upon what she eats during this unique nine-month experience, a woman may either skillfully respond to the changes brought on by the nutritional requirements of pregnancy or make these changes more difficult to handle.

Cultural knowledge and common sense are two of the basic resources we bring to many concerns that arise during pregnancy. If you are a vegetarian, you will probably have acquired vegetarian cultural knowledge on your own and with friends, rather than through relatives and community customs. The importance of common sense is not lost when you have a diet that is not the cultural norm. As you read the information in this book regarding nutrition and the concerns of a vegetarian pregnancy, don't do anything that doesn't feel right to your body. Combine intuition and knowledge for the best results!

I have selected the most common areas in which pregnant vegetarians are likely to voice concerns. Besides providing general information about each particular concern, I have also included recommendations, suggestions for further reading, and some personal experiences of vegetarian moms excerpted from Chapter Two.

If the topic you are looking for is not listed by name below, I encourage you to use the index. Cross-references there will indicate the section which will be most useful in addressing your concern.

Topics Covered in Chapter Three

Physical Health Before Pregnancy

Digestive Changes During Pregnancy

Physical Health During Pregnancy

Vegetarian Diets During Pregnancy

ALLERGIES

One woman wrote to say that she read my first book, *Vegetarian Baby*, not because she was a vegetarian, but because her baby had milk allergies. (*Vegetarian Baby* recommends only minimal dairy products.) Although her husband had had a severe milk allergy as a child, she herself had experienced no such problem so, during her pregnancy, she drank large quantities of milk for the protein.

After she had her baby, she learned that a mother's diet during pregnancy can either oversensitize or desensitize a baby to allergies. It's possible that she created a prenatal environment that made her baby allergic to milk before birth. Avoiding milk during pregnancy might have allowed the baby to be in an allergen-free atmosphere for a longer period, reducing the chances of the allergic response developing at all. Both expectant mothers and fathers who have a family history of allergy are advised either to follow a rotation diet (in which foods containing allergens are eaten less frequently) or to avoid the allergen altogether while the woman is pregnant. In this way, the natural defense systems of the baby can mature without being sensitized by early exposure to potential allergens.

Adele Davis was one of the first people to approach diet holistically and to explain how intricately nutrition and health are linked on the physical, emotional and intellectual levels. She believed that allergies are not irreversible and can be overcome nutritionally. In her view, allergies signal a breakdown of one's ability to digest a particular food. Adequate digestive juices and enzymes in the stomach require a diet with sufficient B vitamins. She suggested adding pantothenic acid (vitamin B_5) as well as vitamin C to increase the rate of growth of intestinal bacteria, which in turn, produce sufficient digestive enzymes to prevent an allergic response.

It is worth checking your families' histories for milk or other food allergies before pregnancy. If obtaining calcium from sources other than milk during pregnancy can help prevent a severe milk allergy in the new baby, it makes sense to find out about the potential for allergy ahead of time so you can make changes in your diet as soon as possible. Lactose is the element in milk that causes intolerance. (See "Milk and Dairy")

Many people have an allergy to wheat. Wheat is a common ingredient in breads, cereals and pastries. While eating whole wheat bread may have seemed like *the* nutritional answer to many people in the '60s, it was not possible for those with wheat allergies. By now every health store and most regular supermarkets stock breads and cereals made from other grains, as well as wheat-free pastas, made from jerusalem artichoke, rice or other plant foods. Quinoa and amaranth, two grain newcomers to the supermarkets, contain no gluten, the most common wheat allergen. This broadening of grain varieties in response to consumer need has made grocery shopping easier and more interesting for vegetarians.

Recommendations

• Remove foods from your diet that are known to cause allergies in close relatives on either side, before pregnancy if possible.

• Consult recipe books that are designed to avoid allergen foods, to be prepared for any dietary changes you might want to make.

Further Information

Note: Most recipe books specifically for people with allergies include meat recipes, but a few are either entirely vegetarian (or vegan) or have a decent vegetarian section.

• *Complete Guide to Food Allergy and Intolerance* by J. Brostoff and L. Gamlin, Crown Publishers, New York, NY, 1992.

• *Freedom from Allergy Cookbook* by Ron Greenberg and Angela Nori, Blue Poppy Press, Vancouver, Canada, 1991. Recipes without wheat, yeast or milk ingredients.

• *McDougall Health Supporting Cookbook, Vol. 1* by the Vegetarian Resource Group, PO Box 1463, Baltimore, MD 21203. Contains wheat-free and dairy-free vegetarian recipes.

• *Wheatless Cooking* by Lynette Coffey, Ten Speed Press, Berkeley, CA, 1985. Mostly non-meat foods: breads, pastries and so on.

• *Whole Way to Allergy Relief and Prevention: A Doctor's Complete Guide to Treatment and Self-Care* by Jacqueline Krohn, Hartley & Marks Publishers, Point Roberts, WA, 1992. Not a cookbook.

• *Taste and See: Allergy Relief Cookbook* by Penny King, Family Health Publications, Sunfield, MI, 1992. Recipes without meat, dairy, eggs, sugar, wheat or vinegar.

ANEMIA

Iron is necessary for our bodies to make and maintain hemoglobin, the protein which transports oxygen in the blood. Iron is stored in hemoglobin, and in another protein, myoglobin, found in the muscles. Anemia is a condition in which there are too few red blood cells or too little total hemoglobin in the blood.

Iron stores are used more rapidly during pregnancy and it is very common for a pregnant woman's body to decrease her available iron. When iron stores are first reduced, there may be no obvious change in how you feel, since the body compensates for a short-term drain. But when hemoglobin production decreases due to a severe reduction in iron stores, you will feel exhausted. Less oxygen is transported by your blood and, as anyone knows who has held her breath, this is tough on the body. Anemia is the most severe result of iron deficiency. An anemic person is more susceptible to illness and also more likely to have pregnancy complications.

In 1988, the American Dietetic Association stated that vegetarians are no more likely to be iron deficient than meat-eaters. Whole grains and legumes, high in iron, are usually lacking in meat-oriented diets. Vegetarians tend to eat more fruit and vitamin C-rich vegetables, increasing their iron absorption by the combination. Vitamin C raises iron efficiency in the body when the two are taken together. (See "Understanding Nutrients: Iron") In fact, vegetarians with good plant food diets are *less* likely to be severely iron-deficient than meat eaters, even during pregnancy.

But since all pregnant women need more iron, an iron supplement is regularly prescribed by doctors, regardless of diet. A reduction in iron level is measurable, but medical nursing manuals call this "pseudoanemia of pregnancy": the total amount of iron and hemoglobin haven't necessarily gone down. Rather the amount of blood has increased to match the needs of pregnancy and so, proportionally, the hemoglobin levels are lower.

Iron is found in two forms: heme and non-heme. Heme iron is found in animal foods and it is relatively easy for the body to absorb. Non-heme iron is primarily found in plant foods. When a person's iron stores are lowered for any reason, non-heme iron becomes more absorbable. A vegetarian diet would thus be able to provide extra usable iron to meet the demands of pregnancy. Before automatically taking a prescribed iron supplement, consider whether it is necessary for you. (See "Supplements")

It is wise to have your iron level checked both before pregnancy and a month or two after conception. The pre-pregnancy count will provide your base, so you know whether you have a low count to start. If so, you may want to increase iron in your diet by eating iron-rich foods right away, before conception. It may not be possible to avoid the natural decrease in iron after pregnancy so starting with a strong iron level means you won't dip too low. Reducing caffeine drinks and aspirin usage before (or during) pregnancy is a complementary approach. This will increase iron absorption from whatever you eat, allowing your hemoglobin to rise to more normal levels.

When your iron level is checked, the result will be expressed either as a number or a percentage. (This measurement is clearly presented in a "Complete Blood Count" table in *Understanding Lab Work in the Childbearing Year,* 4th edition, by Anne Frye, p. 64. This book offers a great deal of practical medical information about pregnancy in language and forms that a lay person can easily understand.) If the number is used, the normal hematocrit level for adult women, up to the 12th week of pregnancy, is 13 to 15 grams of hemoglobin in every 100 milliliters of blood. During the last two months of pregnancy, this falls to an average of 10 to 12 grams per 100 ml. This change is inevitable; the hematocrit level is apparently not raised by additional iron supplements. Since excess iron supplementation is now known to be a health hazard, don't increase your dosage to counteract what is a natural body change.

Hemoglobin carries oxygen for the red blood cells and, expressed as a percentage, is normally 39 to 46 percent of hematocrit for the first part of pregnancy. This percentage naturally falls after the 28th week of pregnancy to a normal range of 30 to 36 percent.

Sometimes a folic acid deficiency rather than an iron deficiency can be the cause of anemia. If increasing iron-rich foods in the diet and taking iron supplements are not effective in raising the hematocrit reading, a folic acid deficiency should be suspected. Blood testing for iron level is routine during any medical care; if you are using a midwife, she should include this in her services. (See "Understanding Nutrients: Folic Acid") Folic acid deficiencies appear to be much more dangerous to healthy development of the fetus, suggesting that prenatal folic acid testing may be even more important than iron testing for the health of both the mother and child.

Anemia is most common in late pregnancy, when the baby's needs are at their height, in addition to the mother's increased nutrient needs. Keep in mind that a slightly lowered iron level is quite normal and let doctors or others know that a vegetarian diet is the most effective remedy for this situation.

Recommendations
• Eat more iron rich foods. Examples: legumes (beans and peas), molasses, wheat germ.

• Combine vitamin C-rich foods with iron-rich foods in your meals.

• Eat lots of iron-rich foods that are also high in vitamin C. Examples: dried fruits, beets and beet greens, chard, spinach, prune juice, grape juice.

• Eat foods rich in copper to increase iron efficiency. Examples: legumes, nuts, dark dried fruits, molasses, avocados, brazil nuts, soybeans.

• Eat foods rich in folic acid. Examples: parsley, chicory, dandelion leaves, watercress, whole grains.

• Cook in iron pots.

• Decrease intake of caffeine (coffee, caffeinated teas, sodas) and tannin (decaffeinated coffees and teas).
• Avoid aspirin because it decreases iron absorption.
• Try deep breathing and yoga as gentle techniques to increase the amount of oxygen in the blood and the efficiency with which it is transported. (See "Exercise")

Further Information

Note: Most information on the topic of anemia is found in medical and research journals, often difficult to obtain except at a good university or college library.

• "Anemias in Pregnancy" by Sue Rodwell Williams, in *Nutrition in Pregnancy and Lactation, 4th Edition*, edited by Bonnie Worthington-Roberts and Sue Rodwell Williams, Mosby Publishing, St. Louis, MO, 1989, pp. 173-177.

• "Anemia vs. Iron Deficiency: increased risk of pre-term delivery in a prospective study" by Theresa School *et al.*, *American Journal of Clinical Nutrition*, 1992, 55:995-998.

• "Coffee consumption as a factor in iron deficiency anemia among pregnant women and their infants in Costa Rica" by Leda Munoz *et al.*, *American Journal of Clinical Nutrition*, 1988, 48:645-651.

• "Protection of maternal iron stores in pregnancy" by L.A. Dawson and W.J. McGanity, *Journal of Reproductive Medicine*, 1988, 32:302-316.

• *Understanding Lab Work in the Childbearing Year, 4th Edition* by Anne Frye, Labrys Press, New Haven, CT, 1990.

Personal Experiences

Kim Pickett-DePaolis

A nurse practitioner suggested that I take iron supplements. I followed her advice and three days later developed a kidney infection. At the same time I happened to be reading Susun Weed's *Wise Woman's Herbal for the Childbearing Years*. She said that iron supplements can cause kidney infections because they are difficult for the kidneys to process and the iron is not absorbed well anyway. She offered a recipe for an iron tonic made from yellow dock root. I took one to two tablespoons a day and my iron count soared! Maybe low iron levels are common for vegetarians during pregnancy, but iron supplements or consuming meat probably hurt more than help.

Linda Tagliaferro
To avoid an iron deficiency, I followed the advice of an acquaintance who was the mother of three children. She recommended a tasty German tonic called Floradix, which has a fabulous fruit flavor and is high in easy-to-assimilate iron. Around my eighth month, I also started taking wheat grass tablets on the advice of another vegetarian mother who had been anemic but cured the problem with them. Because she worried about iron levels, my midwife required frequent blood tests to check my hematocrit. After taking Floradix and wheat grass tablets, I heard those joyous words, "Linda, what are you taking? I want to tell all my other clients! Your hematocrit is so good that I'm going to stop doing blood tests." Balm to my sore fingertips!

Jackie Olson-Newhouse
I had also been anemic for years. When I started drinking beet juice, not only was I not anemic, but I suddenly had lots of energy. Up until that time, it seemed that the first thing on my mind when I woke up each morning was, "When can I squeeze in a nap?"

BLADDER INFECTIONS

Bladder infections (urinary infections) are more common in pregnant women than in non-pregnant women, probably due to hormonal changes that slow the process of urination. When the urine stays inside the body longer, it is more likely to develop the bacteria which produce bladder infections.

The most important prevention and cure is always drinking enough fluids: at least eight glasses a day, especially if you are experiencing a bladder infection. This helps to flush the system by moving fluids along more quickly. With too little water or other healthy liquids, your body will hold onto what fluid it gets and you won't feel as much need to urinate. But urinating at least once an hour is not uncommon during pregnancy; anyone who has been pregnant will sympathize. Besides, it's very important to your health at this time.

Cranberry juice is perhaps the best of fluids to drink to fight an infection that has already started. Eating or drinking citrus fruits and juice will increase the acidity of your urine, inhibiting further bacteria growth.

Be sure to let your medical advisor/doctor know if you have any discomfort during urination since any infection should be monitored. And drink more water and juice whenever you can.

Recommendations
  • Drink at least eight glasses of fluids a day.
  • Drink cranberry juice and/or eat citrus fruits daily.
  • Let your midwife/doctor know about any discomfort during urination.

BODY ACHES AND PAINS

Most body aches and pains during pregnancy are rarely treated nutritionally. In fact, many of these problems are symptoms of mineral deficiencies so it's a good idea to make sure that at least your daily nutritional requirements are being met while you're expecting. Proper exercise and gentle muscle-strengthening exercises will help provide additional support for the body as it adapts to the extra weight and physical changes of pregnancy.

Bone Pains

Although there is not a direct link, the calcium and magnesium demands of the developing baby will reduce calcium and magnesium levels in the mother's blood. Since calcium and magnesium are necessary for healthy bones, an expectant mother needs additional amounts of these minerals, for both herself and her baby. Eating a diet rich in calcium and magnesium, as healthy vegetarians do, will reduce the chance of bone pains and osteoporosis.

The skeletal structure of the body has to shift during pregnancy to make room for the growing baby and its emergence into the world. Bones, particularly the pubic bone, may feel tender during pregnancy.

Recommendations

• Practice Kegel exercises to strengthen the groin muscles. This exercise, which involves contracting and relaxing the muscles used during urination, will help support changes and softening in bones as well as make childbirth easier, with less risk of vaginal tearing due to inflexible muscle tone.

• Practice yoga, especially those postures which stretch and strengthen the lower back muscles. Yoga will help relieve much of the physical discomfort of pregnancy when practiced regularly. (See "Exercise")

• Eat a diet rich in calcium and magnesium from plant foods.

Headaches

Headaches are not a common complaint of pregnancy. If they occur, however, they should be treated with natural remedies rather than aspirin and other synthesized painkillers. Regular exercise is useful in preventing headaches, and active relaxation during stressful times will also reduce this kind of pain.

Migraines are a particularly devastating form of headache that can be triggered by caffeine-rich foods such as chocolate and coffee, as well as by red wines, red meats and many cheeses. Migraine and other headaches are known to be hormonally sensitive and, in women, appear to be frequently associated with a sudden drop in estrogen, which happens during the normal menstrual cycle. But most women who have migraines associated with the menstrual cycle find they disappear during pregnancy, when high levels of estrogen are present.

Prior to the time I got pregnant, I had migraine headaches and required prescription medicine for the severe pain. I was determined not to take this medication during pregnancy, no matter what, although I wondered if my physical response to the pain would affect the baby in its own way. I was relieved and very delighted to discover that, throughout pregnancy, my migraines disappeared completely and only returned when I stopped nursing. If pregnancy does not stop your migraine headaches, be sure to work very closely with a doctor if you feel you require pain medication: all of it reaches the baby. (See "Toxins")

Recommendations

• Make sure you exercise and relax every day, even if that means walking for half an hour during a work break and putting your legs up for half an hour at the end of the day.

• If your migraine headaches do not stop after conception, talk with your midwife/doctor to determine what medicine, if any, might be appropriate.

Muscle Pains and Leg Cramps

The nighttime "charley horse" is common among pregnant women, and some evidence shows that an imbalance between calcium, phosphorus and magnesium may be the cause.

Milk is a high-phosphorus source of calcium. This strong ratio may be a cause of leg cramps, especially if you drink more milk during pregnancy. (See "Milk, Dairy and Eggs") Reducing milk intake and replacing it with other calcium sources that are lower in phosphorus may help the problem.

An alternative is to take calcium supplements to increase the calcium/phosphorus ratio, while continuing to drink milk. The problem is that too much calcium can be a natural abortifacient and, if not monitored, the supplement solution can raise the calcium in the blood and the placenta to a dangerously high level.

Phosphorus intake can be decreased by avoiding processed foods and carbonated drinks, which are phosphorus-rich. In the case of frequent muscle cramps, an additional 20 to 50 mg of magnesium supplement can usually be taken safely, but be sure you don't exceed 300 mg daily in the entire diet.

You may hear this a lot, but only because it is so important. Exercise—stretching the legs and getting the weight off them on a regular basis during pregnancy—will do a lot to prevent muscle cramps. Charley horses may occur mostly at night because that is the time you are most likely to become immobile in an uncomfortable position, reducing free circulation. During later pregnancy, you may find yourself waking more frequently at night: if so, at least stretch your muscles and move around gently in bed. This will encourage good circulation and reduce the chance of cramping after you go back to sleep. (See "Insomnia")

Sometimes, a charley horse cannot be avoided. It rudely wakes you up in the night despite all your precautions and exercise. Try to remember: Never point your toes to relieve the pain. Instead, flex the toes, stretching them up and pushing your heel down. This will begin easing the pain almost immediately. Practice your labor breathing: this practice will be for real and will lessen the pain. Afterwards, rub the area to restore normal circulation.

Recommendations

• Get regular, gentle exercise (walking, yoga, swimming).
• Eat calcium-rich plant foods, such as kale, collards, spinach, chard, broccoli and mustard greens, every day.

CONCEPTION

The process of conception is incredible. Both a woman and a man bring all their genetic and environmental background to the moment of conception. Diet before that moment will determine the healthiness of the sperm, the egg and the ability of the mother's body to nourish a developing baby. Women usually know when they are pregnant, but testing is usually done as verification, as well as to begin a relationship with a midwife/doctor who can help monitor the mother's health throughout her pregnancy.

Formation of Eggs

Eggs begin to develop in the mother's ovaries when she is still developing in her own mother's womb. By the fifth month of her fetal life, all the eggs she will ever produce (around five million) have already been formed. The eggs remain in a premature state in the ovaries until menstruation begins. Then, during each menstruation, an egg matures and is released through the Fallopian tubes, where it may or may not be fertilized. A woman menstruates about 400 times between the onset of her first period and menopause, releasing at least one egg each time. In the ovaries, each egg has its own casing, or follicle. After the egg ripens (about two weeks after the start of the menstrual period), the follicle ruptures, releasing the egg from the ovary into the Fallopian tube where it can be fertilized.

During a woman's life, her eggs are exposed to whatever she is, but with some natural protection by the ovaries. Females are advised to keep x-rays to a minimum and avoid

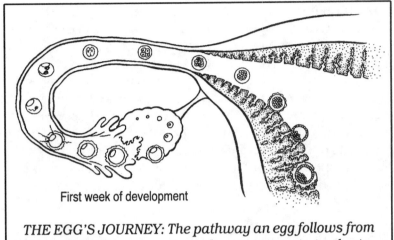

First week of development

THE EGG'S JOURNEY: The pathway an egg follows from its origin in the ovary, through conception, to implantation in the uterine wall.

environmental toxins as much as possible, at least through the childbearing years.

Formation of Sperm

At birth, a boy has immature sperm cells, called spermatogonia. At puberty, boys form the male hormone testosterone in the testicles, which is necessary for the sperm to mature. During the male's life, nearly 1,000 sperm per minute are produced, each about .00024 inch long. This means a man produces about eight trillion sperm over his lifetime! If they're not ejaculated, the sperm are reabsorbed into his body.

Each spermatogonium takes about two months to mature. During this time, it also splits twice, resulting in four mature sperm from each spermatogonium. The sperm must be stored in the testicles, which hang below the body, allowing for a somewhat cooler than body temperature, about 95°F instead of 98.6°F. Higher temperatures can deactivate the sperm. During ejaculation, sperm are gathered (up to 500 million of them) and expelled at a very high speed, about 200 inches per second. An average sperm count is considered to be about 107 million sperm per milliliter of ejaculate.

Since sperm are constantly being created, they are subject to the male's current physical status with their health and survival depending upon the odds in the sheer numbers produced. The sperm that fertilizes an egg will be made by the male about two months earlier. Therefore, it seems wise for a prospective father to be particularly conscious of his diet and health in the several months prior to conception.

Conception

Sperm have a cap containing enzymes which help them remove the outside wall of nutrient cells that surround the ovum. Sperm which make it that far are revived by a glucose bath secreted by the female body. As the sperm remove nutrient layers, the cap dissolves and, finally, one sperm without a cap breaks through the ovum to reach the egg. At this precise moment, the chemical makeup of the ovum rapidly changes, shutting out all other sperm and becoming impenetrable.

How to know if you are pregnant

For most women, the first sign of pregnancy is a missed period. Depending upon how regular your periods are, this sign may be immediate or belated. Depending upon how seriously you are trying to get pregnant, you may or may not consider a late period a sign of pregnancy. In fact, some women do not know they are pregnant for several months, until breast and womb enlargement become physically obvious.

In a second pregnancy, a preliminary sign may be the feeling of letting down milk, as if in preparation for nursing again.

Increased appetite can be another early sign. This is a natural development which encourages the pregnant woman

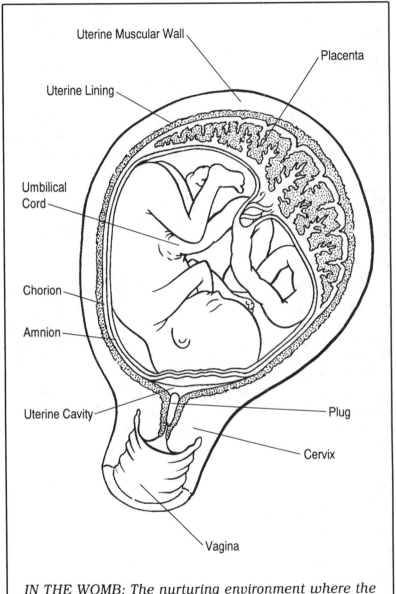

IN THE WOMB: The nurturing environment where the new baby develops.

to eat so that her fetus will have enough nutrients available. In many animals, pregnancy and birth occur during the seasons in which food is most available (spring/summer), adding to the likelihood of the mother being well-nourished. Humans, with their ability to store food artificially, can alter this rhythm.

The placenta functions as the modulator of hormonal changes during pregnancy, balancing the needs of the fetus, which is growing at an enormous rate, and of the mother. The mother's increase in appetite is one response to these internal changes.

Two kinds of tests are used to determine whether a woman is pregnant: urine testing and blood testing.

Urine Tests

Urine strips are now prepared with entirely synthetic chemicals (requiring no rabbit sacrifices). The urine method tests for a placental hormone known as HCG (Human Chorionic Gonadotropin) which rises steadily to a peak between the 60th and 70th day of gestation. Positive results can usually be trusted after the 13th day from the first day a missed period was expected. False results are possible, and may be due to a variety of complicating factors. Simple urine testing supplies are available over the counter at most drugstores.

Such tests can also determine protein, glucose, ascorbic acid, bilirubin and ketone levels in the urine. Establishing a baseline before or in early pregnancy is a good way to keep an eye on health as your pregnancy progresses. This more detailed testing can be done with the purchased, chemically prepared strips which also determine levels of leukocyte, nitrite, pH and blood in the urine. Although not usually included in drugstore pregnancy test kits, these testing strips are available through midwife supply sources such as Moonflower Birthing Supplies, PO Box 128, Louisville, CO 80027.

Blood Tests

Blood testing is far more accurate than urine testing, as well as being valid earlier, but blood testing must be done by registered laboratories. Blood tests also locate HCG in maternal blood serum, and can positively detect pregnancy by the fourth day after the first day of a missed period. However, two-thirds of the time, ectopic pregnancies register as negative results in blood testing.

Further Information

• *A Child is Born* by Lennart Nilsson, Delacorte Press, New York, NY, 1990.

• *At Highest Risk* by Christopher Norwood, Penguin, New York, NY, 1980.

• *Before You Conceive* by John Sussman and Blacke B. Levitt, Bantam Books, New York, NY, 1989.

• "Biologists stumble across new pattern of inheritance" by Gina Kolata, *The New York Times*, July 19, 1991; C-1.

• *Life Before Birth* and *A Time to be Born* by Peter W. Nathanielsz, Promethean Press, NY, 1992.

• "Sperm Wars" by Meredith F. Small, *Discover*, July 1991; 48-53.

• "Tea and Fertility" by A.J. Wilcox and C.R. Weinberg, *Lancet*, 1991, 337:1159-1160.

• *The Midwife's Pregnancy and Childbirth Book* by Marion McCartney and Antonia van der Meer, Harper Perennial, New York, NY, 1991.

• *Understanding Lab Work in the Childbearing Year*, 4th *Edition* by Anne Frye, Labrys Press, New Haven, CT, 1990.

CONSTIPATION

During pregnancy, a mother's body releases the hormone progesterone in greater amounts than usual. Progesterone relaxes the muscles, so that a woman can change shape with additional flexibility. Increasingly relaxed pelvic muscles reduce the chance of vaginal tearing during labor, a pain preventive from Mother Nature.

Progesterone also reduces the efficiency of muscle action in the digestive system. The intestines become sluggish, but process food more completely. This allows the mother's body additional time to extract extra nutrients from food. Simultaneously, the digestive system becomes more efficient at nutrient use, and such important nutrients as calcium and iron become more available.

As a woman's body increases in size during pregnancy, her need for water increases too, both for the amniotic fluid in her womb and for the baby itself. Before pregnancy, a woman needs about 1 ml of water for every kilocalorie of energy used, to keep the fluid levels of the body balanced. During pregnancy, the RDA for water increases by about 30 ml per day, amounting only to about ¼ cup additional water each day. A nursing mother, however, requires about 1,000 ml each day or about one extra quart of liquid per day— don't worry; you'll be thirsty for it! Remember, if you do not drink enough liquid during pregnancy, food can harden as it creeps through the intestine, through lack of moisture.

Consequently, constipation is a clear signal to increase your fluid intake, particularly if it is below eight glasses a day. (Caffeine in sodas, coffees and some teas is a diuretic, so these beverages do not count toward the eight-glass total.) Your body wants you to pay attention to its essential needs, more so with the added needs of a developing baby inside.

During pregnancy the pelvic region shifts position, decreasing the amount of room in the abdominal area. General circulation in that area is slowed by the crowded space. Naturally, the more pregnant you become, the greater the likelihood of constipation, with additional pressure of the growing baby.

Hemorrhoids, the frequently painful swelling of a vein in the anal area, may be aggravated by constipation and the slowing of circulation in the lower digestive tract. Don't try to conquer constipation by straining and pushing—that just increases the pressure in this sensitive area. Instead, try less strenuous efforts, such as those listed below.

Activity, even walking around, is stimulating to the digestive system. If you are not active enough, your intestines can become even more sluggish through the lack of stimulation in their reduced space. Constipation may be a common complaint of pregnancy, but it arises primarily because the digestive system is balanced differently than it is in a non-pregnant body, and we have to adapt to its changing needs.

Although bran foods are often recommended to relieve constipation, they should be eaten with caution during pregnancy. Bran contains phytates and oxalates, both of which bind calcium and remove it from the body before it can be properly absorbed.

Recommendations

• Drink at least eight glasses of water, fruit juice or other healthy liquids every day

• Drink more fruit juice liquids, with pulp if possible. This combines the natural laxative effect of many fruits with additional fluids to soften the stool. Prune juice is a classic remedy, and it provides a lot of iron as well! Fresh pumpkin and squash juice are also healthy laxatives. Warm liquids will help soften stool.

• Dried fruits are good natural laxatives, particularly apricots, raisins, figs and, of course, prunes. Stewed prunes, especially if eaten warm, are easy to digest and very good for you during pregnancy. Don't overdo it with laxative foods, though, because their powerful effect can create gas and other discomfort if your body is not used to the intake.

• Cucumbers, raw greens, molasses, apples and raw sauerkraut are considered laxative foods. Eaten often, they can promote regularity.

• White rice and chocolate may be binding to other foods being digested, increasing the possibility of constipation. High-fiber foods such as bran may help by retaining additional water and keeping stool softer, but they are also more likely to carry calcium out of the system before it can be properly absorbed.

• Don't take laxatives which contain chemicals to activate your digestive system. Metamucil is recommended as one over-the-counter laxative from natural sources that will not harm a fetus.

• Iron supplements are commonly prescribed during pregnancy and, in many diets, a reasonable case can be made for them. However, some forms of iron can be quite constipating. Iron picolinate capsules and liquid iron preparations are preferable.

• Evolve a daily exercise program that is sensitive to the demands of pregnancy. Even though you may keep up your regular exercise program in earlier pregnancy, a natural fatigue may warn you to slow down later. During the third trimester, when heavy physical activity can become too awkward, gentler exercise such as a daily walk or swim can provide the stimulation your digestive system can use to regain its sense of balance.

Personal Experiences
Anonymous

Taking a shit, which I do once or twice a day is a combination of constipation and diarrhea for me—and a wonderful chance to practice my labor lessons. This shit, very black, like well-cooked, mashed black beans (which it may be, at times), comes in cycles within one sitting. I can tell it's in there, but sometimes it seems like if I try to push too hard, I'll push the baby out by mistake.

If I feel stuck when taking a shit, a wonderful technique is rocking my hips and bottom from side to side on the toilet. My intestines start moving things along, threatening to burst out in an explosion on the way. I don't want that to happen, and it frequently makes me wonder if it is similar to labor: I wouldn't want the baby to explode out of me too fast. It would tear me.

So with my body shaking, and tears in my eyes from keeping calm under this pressure, I "pant-blow" to slow it down when it comes out. Then I take a deep breath and relax until I sense another surge from my full intestine. Finally it comes out, without exploding or tearing me apart— what a relief!

After about 10 minutes of this, my intestines are emptied and I'm ready to get on with the rest of being pregnant.

CRAVINGS AND AVERSIONS

No clear evidence indicates that cravings for and aversions to food during pregnancy are either bad or good, as long as the food you answer them with is healthy. Some societies have social taboos on certain foods during pregnancy, providing cultural support for personal aversions.

Food aversions have been described as "definite revulsion for food and drink not previously disliked." A craving is the opposite, a powerful urge toward delicacies for which no previous inordinate desire existed.

At least two-thirds of pregnant women experience cravings and/or aversions, so it is possible to see some patterns among them. A 1978 study of 250 women in New York State showed the foods most frequently craved to be ice cream, sweets, chocolate, fruit and fish. Aversions to foods were found to be more prevalent than cravings; pregnant women in the experiment expressed strong and sudden dislikes of red meat, poultry and sauces containing oregano. In *Nutrition and Metabolism in Pregnancy*, Pedro Rosso also reports that beverages containing caffeine and high-protein foods were the items pregnant women most frequently avoided.

Increased progesterone levels may be responsible for the higher thresholds pregnant women notice in their reactions to salt, sweet, sour and bitter. Cravings and aversions may be the body's way of supplying certain nutrients that might be low or missing from the diet. Late-night hunger should be heeded—you need extra energy, but always try to make the healthiest choice from the foods that appeal to you. A balanced diet taken in regular small amounts will help you differentiate cravings from hunger. During pregnancy, you can expect a natural increase in appetite. Sufficient healthy calories in your diet may help keep the less nutritious cravings (say, for Twinkies) under rational control. You might want to add a strange sweet food at the end of a well-balanced meal, since sugar is far less detrimental in the presence of a full range of nutrients than it is on its own, as a snack.

Carbohydrates

Pregnant women often have an irresistible craving for carbohydrates, particularly less healthy ones such as commercial potato chips and pretzels. This may signal not only a need for additional healthy carbohydrates, but also for sodium, both of which are necessary to the body in greater quantity during pregnancy. Rather than trying to prohibit your indulgence in these empty snack foods, take a look at your overall diet. Eat additional complex-carbohydrate foods: homemade pizza, whole grain breads and cereals. If your diet contains sufficient carbohydrates and protein, snack foods will at least not be used to assuage hunger pangs.

Junk foods are usually highly processed, full of chemicals, lacking in nutrients, wasteful in packaging, and outrageously expensive. Of course you should avoid them, to the best of your ability. But fighting the desire for such foods is rarely effective directly and often leads to a sense of frustration and guilt over lack of control. If you have a healthy diet, the detrimental effects of junk foods will be kept to a minimum.

Dairy products

Although meat is commonly found to be distasteful during pregnancy, dairy products, particularly milk, are often craved. Consumed in quantity during pregnancy, milk may have a calcium/phosphorus ratio that can upset the balance of your system. (See "Body Aches and Pains") If you drink milk, keep the amounts to a reasonable level so that your calcium intake is not far above the required amount. (See "Milk and Dairy Products" and "Understanding Nutrients: Calcium")

Ice

A persistent craving for ice is considered a possible indicator of anemia. Since it is a well-documented craving, be sure your iron level is adequate.

Meat

Some vegetarian women crave red meat during pregnancy; many others find an even stronger aversion than before. If you do crave meat, it will probably be something you particularly liked during childhood, as many psychological factors operate during pregnancy to cause you to seek out comforting foods. One pregnant strict vegetarian found herself unable to resist fresh venison at a friend's picnic, despite her own surprise. If you do feel an uncontrollable urge to eat meat, keep it to a minimum and eat only organically raised meats.

Aversions to meat are far more common than cravings for meat during pregnancy. Many cultures have had taboos against eating meat during pregnancy. Meats are harder to digest, more likely to hold toxins and rot sooner than vegetable foods, so this widespread aversion could easily have biological roots, protecting the fetus from a food that is unlikely to be healthy. (See "Meat and Meat Hazards")

Pica

Pica is a strange and unhealthy craving for non-food substances such as laundry starch or clay. It has been observed throughout the world, but most frequently among pregnant women and malnourished children. Clay contains nutrients such as calcium, iron and magnesium, although there is some question as to whether they are in a form that humans can use. Some indications show that pica may be a symptom of an iron deficiency, but evidence for this has not been clearly established. In fact, pica may turn out to contribute to an iron deficiency rather than result from it.

A 1991 article in *The Sciences* magazine discusses the most prevalent form of pica—eating clay, or geophagy. Author Timothy Johns suggests that clay-eating is not as strange a custom as one might think. Clay detoxifies and reduces the bitterness of tannins found in some acorns and potatoes. In areas such as the Andes, green potatoes are dipped into a clay and water sauce before being eaten, providing a tolerable taste when only green potatoes are available to eat. In places where healthy food is scarce and available food is not very edible, clay has turned out to be a natural aid to digestion by reducing astringent tastes and resultant nausea.

According to Johns, "Novel foods can be of unpredictable quality; it is impossible to tell just by looking at them whether they are safe to eat. Fortunately, people and other animals have various physiological and behavioral mechanisms for dealing with toxins. Nausea and vomiting are obvious examples: both mechanisms quickly remove offending foods from the gastrointestinal tract, thereby preventing toxins from being absorbed into the body. They also warn the consumer—rather harshly—not to eat more of the food. Not surprisingly, toxins are the main line of defense for many plants. Clay-eating appears to be a similar mechanism in that it allows animals to make their way through an uncertain and potentially threatening dietary environment. . . . Clay-eating thus persisted as a kind of buffer, or protective device, for quelling gastrointestinal stress induced by barely tolerable wild plants or pangs of hunger . . . the adoption of geophagy as a general response to toxins allowed people to make wider use of natural resources."

If clay is good for digestion, then it is not quite so surprising that pregnant women might be drawn to eating clay on some biological level—the nausea of pregnancy is widespread enough to transcend time and geography. In Zambia, a clay is sold as a stomach medicine, primarily to pregnant women. Nor is modern society ignoring this ancient wisdom: Johns points out in his article that Kaopectate contains kaolinite, an active element in the Zambian clay.

But is it healthy for pregnant women eat clay as a cure for nausea? Unfortunately, clay is rarely free of more dangerous elements such as lead. Clay in excess can harm the digestive system and may reduce the appetite through a feeling of fullness without contributing a proportional nutritive value. Therefore, it should be avoided. If you notice yourself having cravings of this nature, make sure you are eating a nutrient-rich, well-balanced diet, and give in to other healthier cravings first.

Sweets
During pregnancy, your need for additional protein increases by approximately 15 percent. Pregnant or not, a lack of protein in the diet will frequently result in a craving for sweets, and so such a craving may be counterbalanced by increasing protein and complex carbohydrate intake. Sweets can be eaten in moderation, but should never be used as an answer to hunger pangs.

Further Information

• *Nutrition and Metabolism in Pregnancy* by Pedro Rosso, Oxford University Press, New York, NY, 1990.

• *Nutrition in Pregnancy and Lactation* by Bonnie S. Worthington-Roberts and Sue Rodwell Williams, eds.; C.V. Mosby Co., St. Louis, MO, 1989.

• *Pickles and Ice Cream* by Mary Abbott Hess and Anne Elise Hunt, McGraw-Hill Book Co., New York, NY, 1982.

• "Well-Grounded Diet: The Curious Practice of Eating Clay is Rooted in Its Medicinal Value" by Timothy Johns, *The Sciences*, Sep/Oct 91:38-43.

Personal Experiences

Gayle Brandeis

When certain foods began to turn my stomach, I suspected I was pregnant. A test confirmed my instinct. The next morning, after two years of veganhood, I ordered eggs for breakfast. I cannot really explain why I chose to begin eating eggs and dairy products again. I know it is perfectly possible to have a successful vegan pregnancy, but somehow it felt right to return to a lacto-ovo lifestyle. Perhaps I was influenced by subconscious connections, my mind linking egg with womb, milk with breast. Perhaps I didn't trust my personal vegan protein consumption. Whatever the cause, I'm grateful I trusted my intuition about my diet, for I had a glowingly healthy pregnancy.

Faye Lilyerd

My husband and I adopted the "Fit for Life" eating style in 1987, after reading the books written by Harvey and Marilyn Diamond. On average, I ate fruit until noon, a salad for lunch, and heavier foods at supper. I was also drinking a fresh glass of carrot-apple-beet juice in the morning, until I realized I was two months pregnant.

Light morning sickness started at that time, and I couldn't keep juice down. The sight of fruit made me nauseous. I ate cereal and toast for breakfast, using nutmilks and soymilk. Fresh vegetables still appealed to me. My nausea lasted only a month, but my tolerance for fruits stayed low, only about half of what I was used to.

Valerie Schultz

During my first trimester, I wildly craved yogurt. Even though my head knew a vegan pregnancy was perfectly viable, my nerves gave into my doubts. I started eating yogurt at least once a day for the rest of my pregnancy.

Another dietary change during pregnancy involved beans. I had embraced the poetry in the image of the pot of beans soaking in my kitchen: sorting and soaking different varieties of beans had become an almost daily family ritual. But during the first three months of this pregnancy, I could barely stand the thought of beans. One night I cooked up a batch of Portuguese Beans—a family favorite—and burst into tears at the sight of them steaming in my bowl. A long while passed before I ate beans again. And even then I started small—with lentils.

Kiana Dicker

I believe in letting the body tell you what it wants—and then researching the validity of that desire. My inclination was to eat lightly and often, downing gallons of raspberry leaf tea and watered-down juices. Ginger tea and frequent handfuls of mixed nuts, dried fruit and figs banished all signs of morning sickness which had nagged at my peace of mind in the early months. Throughout my pregnancy I lived with a greasy sensation in my mouth. I longed for licorice, which, although normally good for women, can be an abortifacient for a pregnant one. I could down six boxes of mint TicTacs in one sitting—not good. Buckets of iced mint tea and chomping on mint leaves helped me avoid that. I also swathed myself in a highly aromatic aromatherapy cream. I really wanted to eat it, but smelling it calmed the irrational urge.

Valerie Taylor

I had a strange and irresistible craving for fish sticks with tartar sauce when I was pregnant. I had never craved fish sticks before pregnancy. When I finally gave in, they tasted as good as I was thinking they would! I went through a period when I had them at least once a week even though I don't really consider them food. But they sure were good at the time.

Lonna Wilkinson

During the first trimester of my pregnancy, I noticed several changes in my food desires. I soon found I was eating eggs and dairy in greater amounts than before. This seemed to be the simplest and most satisfying way to meet my body's demands for protein. Strangely, foods that I normally avoided and considered to be greasy, salty or processed suddenly caught my eye. At work, I was amazed to find myself drooling over the university cafeteria food and to find that pizza, Fritos and other vending machine snacks seemed irresistible. My interest in salt was at an all-time high, but I did not desire sweets or sugar at all. The only aversion I ever developed was for Mexican foods, which was surprising because it is usually standard fare in our house.

DETOXIFICATION

While some cleansing procedures can be done before you are pregnant, most are not recommended after conception. For example, fasting is one common way to get rid of toxins. But if you are fasting, you aren't getting any nutrients, which a fetus needs on a steady basis to develop into a healthy baby. If your pregnant body has good nutrition reserves to start, you will probably experience no adverse effects from a brief fast—but neither will you benefit. If you fast to cleanse an unhealthy body without stores of nutrients in place for back-up, fetal development may suffer.

But if you have a chance to fast before you get pregnant, you may want to take the opportunity. Check with your doctor or medical advisor before starting a fast, to make sure you have no complicating factors such as high blood pressure or hypoglycemia.

Usually, three days is considered the minimum time to fast if you are trying to clean your body of toxins. Often fasting includes drinking teas or juices; water should always be available to avoid dehydration. You may feel temporarily weakened as the toxins leave your body, but that is common. Sometimes people get sick from fasting; should that happen to you, consult your medical advisor if you decide to continue.

Herbs such as yarrow, echinacea, elder root, rosemary and golden seal have been used as cleansing herbs; they are usually taken during a fast or cleansing period, but not on a regular basis since they are quite potent. If you are unfamiliar with these herbs, be sure to talk to someone knowledgeable before using them to detoxify your body. Do *not* use them after conception as they may cause miscarriage.

After conception, fasting is rarely a good idea. Instead, good nutrition offers the best protection for the fetus, while also healing your body from toxic invasions of the past. Foods that are high in vitamin C, vitamin E and beta carotene will naturally fortify and protect your system against environmental hazards such as pollution and mild exposure to radiation.

While it is not true for everyone, if you are already a vegetarian it is likely that you will have already begun to clear your personal environment of toxins that can be particularly harmful during pregnancy. For example, fewer vegetarians smoke cigarettes than non-vegetarians, so a warning about the dangers of smoking may be relatively unnecessary in a book on vegetarian pregnancies. However, if you do smoke, you should make a concerted effort to stop at least six months before getting pregnant to allow your body time to clean out tobacco-related toxins. If your partner or other housemates smoke, make sure that common areas such as kitchens, bathrooms and living rooms are smoke-free. Passive smoking (or breathing smoke-filled air) can be just about as harmful as smoking yourself.

Recommendations

• If you are planning to get pregnant, give up as many "vices" (cigarettes, alcohol, caffeine and so on) as you can at least three to six months before conception. That way, you can cleanse your system and go through the difficulty of giving up unhealthy addictions before your body concentrates on pregnancy. Withdrawal is not always easy, but it is better not to overload your body with changes in habits at the same time you are trying to conceive.

• Fast before conception, not afterwards: your body needs the nutrients during pregnancy to prepare itself for the process of creating and growing a new human being. After fasting, be sure to eat well to rebuild stores of nutrients that may have been lost through the fast or other detoxification procedures.

• Foods like carrots, broccoli, green leafy vegetables (mustard greens, kale, chard, beet greens and the like), and cantaloupe offer plentiful vitamin C and beta carotene. Vitamin E can be found in wheat germ, whole grain breads and cereals and legumes. Try to eat lots of fresh, organically produced fruits and vegetables to keep your immune system at its healthiest.

• Fruit juice, particularly cranberry and blueberry juice, has been shown to inhibit vaginal and urinary tract infections, according to reports in *The New England Journal of Medicine*, so drink these juices plentifully.

• Aerobic exercise will eliminate stored toxins such as DDT and PCBs, which can prevent a full-term pregnancy if levels within the mother's body are too high. Start aerobic exercise before pregnancy, since it is a strenuous exercise that is not easy on the body if you are not used to it. (See "Exercise") Additionally, you will want to get rid of toxins before conception since an intense loss of toxins will result in a higher percentage being sent to the placenta as they are released from storage in the mother's body.

• Pregnancy itself often produces some natural aversions to things that may harm the fetus: caffeine, alcohol and cigarettes may be particularly unpleasant during these nine months. If you haven't been able to give up unhealthy habits before conception, you will find these internally produced aversions quite helpful in increasing your willpower! (See "Cravings and Aversions")

DIGESTION

Because an expectant woman's body creates and feeds another being, nutritional requirements change drastically during pregnancy. From taste buds to intestines, the digestive system also changes in order to meet these needs. The placenta is a primary regulatory mechanism during pregnancy, responsible for increasing the output of hormones that signal hunger and spark the appetite of the mother.

During pregnancy, many women notice a change in their appetite, but this varies from person to person. Some women are always hungry from the earliest months of pregnancy, but many others experience a drop in appetite due to nausea or morning sickness, common in the first trimester. Almost all women experience a major increase in appetite during the second trimester, followed by a reduction during the third trimester. Then the stomach's space is cramped and a sensation of fullness occurs even with less food.

An appetite increase is a natural way of assuring that the mother eats enough to support her own healthy functioning

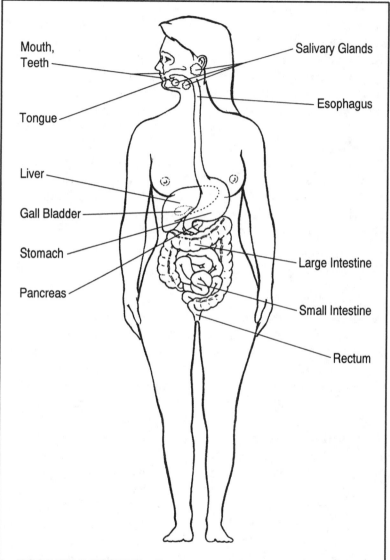

FOOD PROCESSING: From taste buds to intestines, the digestive system changes to meet the nutritional needs of pregnancy.

as well as the proper nutrition of the fetus. In animals, pregnancy and birth often occur during the seasons in which food is most available (spring/summer), adding to the likelihood of a well-nourished mother and child. Through refrigeration and packaging, humans have the ability to store food artificially, which may complement seasonal changes in appetite but, considering the degree to which human life may deviate from Nature's rhythms, may also counteract proper nourishment.

It's easy to observe seasonal variations in food intake. People, particularly in the temperate zones, are likely to eat less during summer and more heartily during the winter. Soups and baked foods, for example, warm kitchen and stomach in the winter but during the summer, hot foods are far less appealing. Even using the stove and oven in hot weather can add to the unpleasant heat and result in a reluctance to cook hearty meals. Adele Davis, purveyor of some dietary overreaction, suggests that fetuses carried during extremely hot summer months are more likely to be smaller at birth, with a higher incidence of complications as a result. Eating well during hot weather is an important challenge.

In addition to the natural increase in appetite a woman may experience during pregnancy, her body also becomes far more efficient in absorbing and utilizing vitamins and minerals. The entire digestive process slows down so that foods remain in the stomach and intestines longer. In this way, the body has more time to assimilate nutrients, and uses up less energy in the process. An increase in stomach acid processes nutrients more completely, and essential elements such as iron, B vitamins and protein are extracted in higher percentages. In effect, the nutrients become more available during pregnancy (See "Understanding Nutrients: Iron, B Vitamins, Protein")

Digestive problems of one sort or another are common during pregnancy, because of this slowing of digestion. Extra stomach acid can produce a variety of uncomfortable side

effects, such as nausea, heartburn, constipation and flatulence. (See individual entries for more information.) A vegetarian diet rich in well-chewed raw foods will go a long way
toward eliminating the most harmful of these symptoms—
constipation.

Pregnancy is not the time to switch from a meat-centered
diet to a vegan diet: any radical dietary change is not easy
for your body to handle on top of pregnancy. It takes a while
to adapt from eating high-protein, high-fat animal foods to
eating grains and legumes. It takes a while for your body to
become cleansed and efficient at absorbing nutrients. A
radical change of diet could mean reduced nutrient availability for a while, not to mention digestive discomforts such
as gas. A far gentler and more reasonable approach is to
change your diet before pregnancy, gradually reducing animal foods and replacing them with grains, vegetables and
legumes at the center of meals. Rudolf Ballantine's book,
Transition to Vegetarianism, is one of the most helpful guides
in this process.

Recommendations

• Chew slowly and thoroughly. The teeth break food
into mush and saliva is designed to do a great deal of digesting before food even reaches your stomach. The more completely you chew, the more nutrients you will get from your
food and the less likely you will be to experience indigestion.

• Eat small, frequent meals as the best preventive measure in keeping your body's digestive challenges within a
comfortable range.

• Regular gentle exercise is *essential* in regulating and
toning the digestive system.

• Foods such as avocados, bananas, mangoes, sprouts,
papaya and pineapples are rich in enzymes that are active
in digestion.

• Be aware of the changes in your digestive system due
to pregnancy and treat them with respect: they are respon-

sible for the way a healthy baby is nourished. A slower digestion process may be frustrating but if you accept the new
rhythm, it will be easier and healthier for you and your baby.

• Eat a well-balanced diet, no matter what the level of
your appetite or food intake. Don't stuff yourself and don't
starve yourself.

Further Information

• "The iron and zinc status of long-term vegetarian
women" by B.M. Anderson *et al.*, *American Journal of Clinical Nutrition*, 1981, 34:1042-1048.

• "Trace element status in healthy subjects switching
from a mixed to a lactovegetarian diet for 12 months" by
T.S. Srikumar *et al.*, *American Journal of Clinical Nutrition*,
1992, 55:885-890.

• *Transition to Vegetarianism* by Rudolph Ballentine, The
Himalayan Institute, Honesdale, PA, 1987.

EDEMA (FLUID RETENTION)

During the last trimester of pregnancy, it is common for
a woman's hands and ankles to become slightly swollen. This
is normal if it is a mild swelling only; extra fluids in your body
may collect if you stand for a long time because of the baby's
weight at the top of your legs. As a result of this pressure,
additional fluid may be displaced from the abdomen and
pushed downwards. As circulation slows at the top of your
leg, gravity will force any extra fluid out to your extremities—
ankles and hands. This is a hint to get off your feet more
frequently to relieve the pressure and allow more normal
circulation.

Sudden or severe swelling may be a symptom of toxemia, especially when blood pressure is high and/or a urine
sample shows a rise in protein level. Swelling in the hands

or face are more of a concern than swollen ankles. If edema should suddenly occur or increase, or if swelling starts in your arms, be sure to contact your midwife/doctor as soon as possible. (See "High Blood Pressure, Toxemia")

Recommendations

• Be sure to give your feet and legs a rest every day by elevating them above the level of your chest (reclining or prone position). This will help prevent as well as reduce edema by increasing proper circulation.

• Do not restrict fluids or salt to compensate for swelling—that will only upset the sodium/fluid balance of your body even more. For the same reason, do not take diuretics.

• Alert your medical advisor/doctor if you are experiencing edema.

• Be sure you are eating sufficient protein, about 60 grams a day. Protein acts like a diuretic to a certain extent, drawing in fluid, with excess excreted through the kidneys. But remember that overdoing protein intake can cause a calcium imbalance in the system, particularly if you are not using milk or other dairy products.

• Promptly check with your midwife/doctor about any sudden or extensive swelling.

Further Information

• *The Midwife's Pregnancy and Childbirth Book* by Marion McCartney and Antonia van der Meer, Harper Perennial, New York, NY, 1991.

EGGS

Like milk, eggs are often rumored to be a perfectly balanced protein food and, for this reason, are often recommended to pregnant women. While their protein profile is indeed ideal, eggs bring up so many potential concerns that they seem like a less than healthy suggestion.

Poultry farms are notorious for high-chemical feed. Eggs can contain pesticides, growth hormones, antibiotics and bacteria that were present in the hen that laid them. Salmonella is the most common bacteria, infecting about one-third of raw chicken in the United States, according to the USDA. In humans, salmonella poisoning is severe and comes from eating contaminated eggs in a raw or partially cooked condition, which can be the case in ice cream, mayonnaise, some salad dressings and very softly boiled eggs.

The growing fetus is even more at risk from salmonella, so pregnant women should be careful to avoid raw or partially cooked eggs altogether. If you use eggs, look for ones from hens which have been raised without pesticides or antibiotics. Buy only fresh eggs and store them immediately in a refrigerator since salmonella breeds rapidly at room temperature. Do not use cracked eggs, or eggs over three weeks old. Raising a chicken yourself may be the best way to have fresh eggs free of contaminants; with only one chicken, your egg intake will also be naturally limited.

Egg yolks are very high in cholesterol. Although the lecithin in egg whites may provide a balance, it does not completely counteract the yolk's effects. Since one large egg provides the recommended daily maximum of cholesterol, it is easy to see how cholesterol blood levels can be raised by eating the ideal American diet of the '50s (and '60s, '70s and '80s?): two eggs, bacon, toast with butter, milk and juice.

As with milk, dairy and meat, eggs are a concentrated but unnecessary protein source. Protein from beans, tofu and a balanced vegan diet based on one of several dietary plans will provide plenty of protein without risking exposure to the hazards of eating animal products. (See "Food Groups, Dietary Plans and RDAs")

Further reading
 • *Safe Food: Eating Wisely in a Risky World* by Michael F. Jacobson, Living Planet Press, Venice, CA, 1991 (especially Chapter 4: "Meat, Poultry and Eggs").
 • *The A to Z Guide of Toxic Foods and How to Avoid Them* by Lynn Sonberg, Pocket Books, New York, NY, 1992.

EXERCISE

Exercise makes me think of exhausting workouts. But some exercise is essential for proper assimilation of nutrients. With regular activity, your body will absorb vitamins and minerals in greater amounts and with greater efficiency. During pregnancy, a good deal of your nutrition is going to help the baby grow inside you, but some physical activity on a regular basis is good for all the systems of your body: circulatory, hormonal, nervous, cardiovascular. The way you get exercise will change over the nine-month period you are pregnant to allow more of your energy to go to the baby. I have known runners to continue their daily regimens far into pregnancy, but even the most devoted exerciser will eventually hear her body say, "Take it easy."

Exercise keeps oxygen flowing freely in the blood, toning the muscles so that the blood can more easily carry nutrients to all parts of the mother's body, as well as to the placenta and, ultimately, the baby. A fit body is better able to handle the changes of pregnancy, the physical stresses of labor and the restoration of the body to its pre-pregnancy form after birth. *The American Journal of Obstetrics and Gynecology* reported that women who exercise regularly during pregnancy are likely to have shorter labors, less need for physical intervention, and fewer caesareans.

Aerobic exercises are fine for early pregnancy *only* if you are used to them. Aerobics provide a good cleansing of the body before pregnancy, eliminating stores of toxins, like DDT and PCBs. Since the toxins may circulate in the body before being eliminated, it is important to *begin* an intense aerobics program or to use a detoxification diet only before you conceive, never once you are pregnant. (See "Detoxification")

Pre-conception is also a good time to give special attention to strengthening muscles which will be affected by pregnancy, in the abdomen, lower back and pelvis. Toning in advance allows your body to function at peak performance during pregnancy.

Running or jogging can be continued as long as you feel comfortable with this level of activity. Keep in mind that pregnancy is not the time to overstress. If you feel your body resisting a normal level of exercise, trust what you feel and slow down a little. During vigorous physical activity, the rate of blood flow is altered to supply the body with extra energy. The increase in blood flow decreases blood supply to the placenta, and fewer vitamins and minerals are available to the growing baby. This is not harmful in the short term, but continued overstressing will ultimately affect fetal development.

Taking it easy does not mean sitting a lot. Besides, extended sitting will (most likely) make you feel uncomfortable: you *need* to get some physical activity on a regular basis for proper digestion. Even if you are just moving from room to room, the activation of your physical body will help your food be properly digested. Although this may sound simplistic, it is true.

Even gentle exercise and deep breathing will energize you when you feel dragged out and, in many ways, the age-old wisdom of yoga prevails during pregnancy: Don't strain anything, but keep moving.

Recommendations

• Try hatha yoga. Probably because I grew up during the '60s, this was my preferred form of exercise during pregnancy. Not only was it calming at a time when my moods seemed to swing a lot, but it helped to strengthen many muscles involved in pregnancy without requiring vigorous exercise. (See "Yoga" for some of the yoga postures I used during pregnancy.) Yoga involves deep breathing, which carries extra oxygen throughout the body in the blood, giving your whole body and baby a healthy treat: fresh oxygen! Yoga can be done on your own or with a class; in my town, the YMCA offered a yoga class for pregnant women. (By the way, I think women who take yoga classes may be likely to be pro-vegetarian, providing a common bond if it is missing elsewhere in your environment.)

• Swimming is another good form of exercise during the pregnancy months because it reduces the weight of your body for a while. Everything feels more comfortable with (comfortably warm) water around you. Many larger hotels often offer public swimming hours for a small fee, as do fitness centers and high school pools. (For example, where I live, public swimming hours are available at the Holiday Inn and the Sheraton, as well as at the YMCA.) I hear that hotel pools are usually comfortably warm.

• Walking is the most convenient form of exercise for many busy pregnant women. Walking to and from work, going on errands that involve walking, and walking for pleasure are all ways to get regular exercise. Walking should always be combined with resting in a semi-inverted position (feet above chest level) to take the pressure off your lower body, reduce the incidence of edema or swelling in your ankles. (See "Edema")

• Don't eat and walk at the same time, even to save time. Eating requires a (relatively) still body for food to be digested properly and nutrients absorbed well. And don't exercise to the point of dehydration. Sufficient water is vital during pregnancy.

• Join a prenatal exercise classes. I joined my YMCA class during my sixth month of pregnancy. It met twice a week for about 45 minutes, with about 20 women in all stages of pregnancy. Although it was fun to get together with other mothers, the teacher had never been pregnant and it showed. For example, when she sat up, she sat straight up from a lying-down position. The preferred method of sitting up for pregnant women is rolling to one side and using your arms to push you up. This puts less stress on the abdomen and lower back muscles, particularly in later pregnancy. But I stayed in the class and, as I started to exercise more regularly, my general energy level rose and it was easier to be active. One of the telling signs of a good exercise class is how you feel afterwards—I always felt great, as did my classmates, no matter how pregnant they were. If you have a choice (I had none), I would recommend finding a teacher who has been pregnant, and I would recommend going to such a class if you have time, because the camaraderie is wonderful. Being around a lot of energetic pregnant women is very inspiring.

• If you were a regular jogger before pregnancy, you can continue, but be sure to wear good running shoes and stay away from concrete or paved surfaces, to protect your joints. If you want to continue to attend aerobics classes, make sure you go to a low-impact class for less wear and tear on the joints and ligaments; they're already getting plenty of encouragement to stretch from your pregnancy. Be sure to drink plenty of liquids before and after exercise to prevent dehydration.

• Stretch your legs: Before getting up in the morning, rotate your feet gently to increase circulation. Don't point your toes to stretch your legs as this may start a leg cramp. If you feel a leg cramp starting, point your toes towards your knees rather than out straight; this will reduce the pain much faster. Your inclination may be to stretch your feet away from your body, but this will only make the cramp worse. Flexing your foot the other way can stop it.

• To tie your shoes or put on socks, put your foot up on a chair, bringing it closer to your hands rather than bending

---

Guidelines for Exercise During Pregnancy
From the American College of Obstetricians and Gynecologists

1. Drink plenty of fluids before, after and, if necessary, during exercise.

2. Avoid exercise during hot, humid weather or when feverish.

3. Keep your maximum heart rate between 130 and 140 beats per minute, depending upon your age. For a more exact suggested maximum rate for you, ask your obstetrician.

4. Do not exercise strenuously for longer than 15 minutes during any one session.

5. Avoid any exercise that is performed lying on the back after the completion of the fourth month.

6. Avoid jerky, bouncy movements, as well as either deep flexion or extension of the joints.

7. Include five-minute warm-up and cool-down periods in your exercise routine.

8. Exercise regularly—at least three times a week—rather than sporadically.

---

over. If you have to reach something on the floor, squat while keeping your back straight. Not only does this protect the lower back muscles, but squatting is excellent for toning the pelvic muscles and the thighs.

• Walking around: Try to be aware of your posture, making sure your back is straight and your pelvis is tucked in. The natural tendency is to let your abdomen pull forward with your buttocks compensating, but a swayback position will quickly cause back aches and weaken abdominal muscles. This is particularly important if you are carrying something like groceries. Try walking smoothly and perhaps even a little more slowly, and don't forget to breathe!

Further Information
• *Moving through Pregnancy* by Elisabeth Bing, Macmillan Books, New York, NY, 1975.
• *The Complete Pregnancy Exercise Book* by Diane Simkin, New American Library, New York, NY, 1980.
• *Essential Exercises for the Childbearing Year* by Elizabeth Noble, Houghton Mifflin Co., Boston, MA, 1988.

FLATULENCE

Flatulence, or intestinal gas, is a by-product of the digestive action of bacteria that live in the large intestine. When sugar, starches and fiber reach the large intestine without being digested enough, these bacteria produce gas. Complex-carbohydrate foods most likely to produce gas are beans, onions, dried fruits, Brussels sprouts, cabbage and broccoli.

Most people experience flatulence and gas pains, although the digestive changes of pregnancy may make them more likely during this time. (See "Constipation " and "Nausea")

Recommendations
• Eat slowly and chew well. These are the best preventive measures for flatulence. Particularly with complex carbohydrates, the more digestive juices that are applied at the beginning of the digestive cycle—in the mouth—the easier the food will be to digest when it reaches your stomach.
• Be aware of which foods make you feel gassy and chew these foods an extra ten times per mouthful or prepare them in a more easily digestible way. For example, broccoli is an extraordinarily nutritious food that you may prefer to continue eating even though it sometimes causes gas. Broccoli soup is a good alternative to eating raw or lightly cooked broccoli during pregnancy.
• If you are not used to eating beans frequently in your diet, only include them in small quantities until your sys-

tem gets used to them. Many people find that their bodies become accustomed to beans over time and no longer have gas problems but, for others, the flatulence they connect to beans may have inhibited them from eating beans long enough to become acclimated.

• Here are several recommendations for reducing the gas-producing qualities of beans: pre-soak beans, cook them for a longer time over a lower heat, add a piece of the sea-vegetable kombu or a bay leaf to beans before and/or during cooking. Beano is a popular product sold at most health food stores and manufactured by AkPharma Inc., PO Box 111, Pleasantville, NJ 08232-0111. It is a liquid enzyme product that breaks down raffinose, one of the primary complex sugars found in beans that is known to produce gas. Up to eight drops with your first bite of food will supposedly add a sufficient amount of the enzyme alpha-galactosidase to reduce gas when eating beans and other raffinose-rich products. The enzyme comes from a mold called *Aspergillus niger*, "derived from food-grade fungal sources" and on the FDA's "Generally Recognized As Safe" list. It appears to work, judging from testimonials, although I personally haven't tried it. It has not been tested on pregnant women.

• Slippery elm bark tea has been known to soothe digestive problems and absorb intestinal gases.

FOOD COMBINING

Food combining is a way of working with the digestive process rather than against it as we plan our meals and snacks. All societies have cultural food combinations that occur as regionally produced foods form the basis of daily recipes. Most of these recipes have supported life over many centuries and so it is no surprise that many of them use principles of food combining to increase protein availability and overall digestibility.

In 1951, Dr. Herbert M. Shelton published *Food Combining Made Easy*, still the current standard reference on the topic. Shelton incorporated his knowledge and experience to offer a written plan for reducing digestive problems which cause discomfort and illness. He believed that once a child is weaned from its mother, milk is no longer a particularly healthy food. Because of the length of time it takes to digest flesh foods, he cautioned against animal products, which are such highly concentrated protein sources.

Although Shelton's theories are often disregarded by nutritionists and researchers, they certainly will cause no harm. Pregnant women should be encouraged to snack on fruits instead of junk foods, and so eating oranges, strawberries or orange juice between meals rather than with them may be more appealing in many ways. Sometimes a combination of foods may seem distasteful to a pregnant women whereas eating foods individually will not have the same effect. (See "Sensory Changes")

Shelton understood before Frances Moore Lappé that proteins need not be combined in the same meal to provide balanced amino acids (see "Protein Complementing" and "Understanding Nutrients: Protein"). He actually suggested that proteins should *never* be combined. Other meal combinations he considers detrimental to digestion are:

- Acid/starch combinations, such as fruits on cereals
- Protein/starch combinations, such as meat and potatoes
- Protein/protein combinations, such as milk and anything else
- Protein/acid combinations, such as fruit juices with bean soup
- Protein/sugar combinations, such as desserts with dinner
- Sugar/starch combinations, such as sweet rolls
- Acid fruits or melons with anything else (including each other)

For a person who eats flesh foods, these guidelines begin to look pretty strange as they translate into meal times: a series of eight to ten meals a day of single foods might be the only way to conform to this regimen on a meat-centered diet. However, Shelton believes that non-starchy and green vegetables combine well with anything, including proteins such as legumes, nuts and seeds. For vegetarians, Shelton's method of food combining has far fewer restrictions:

- Eat acid fruits alone (tomatoes can be combined with non-starchy vegetables, nuts, or avocado)
- Eat melons alone
- Avoid oily salad dressings

Additionally, since digestion is slowed during pregnancy (See "Digestion" and "Constipation"), following some of Shelton's principles of food combining may be helpful in allowing digestion of individual foods to be concentrated and thus more efficient. For specific food combination lists and recipes, consult the references recommended below.

Further Information
- *Food Combining for Vegetarians* by Jackie Le Tissier, Thorsons Publishers, London, England, 1992.
- *Food Combining Made Easy* by Herbert M. Shelton, Willow Publishing, San Antonio, TX, 1982.
- *Food Combining Simplified, 3rd Revised Edition* by Dennis Nelson, self-published, 1988. Order from: D. Nelson, PO Box 2302, Santa Cruz, CA 95063.

FOOD GROUPS, DIETARY PLANS AND RDAs

Food groups and dietary plans are usually based upon nationally accepted recommended dietary allowances (commonly known as the RDAs). In the United States, the RDAs have been determined by the Food and Nutrition Board of the National Research Council since 1941. The most recent recommendations, the 10th edition of the RDAs, were published in 1989. The RDAs of each nutrient are given in Chapter Four.

Recommendations are changed for a number of reasons. As science learns more about the interactions of nutrition and human development, age groupings have changed. For example, since the 1980 RDAs, it has been discovered that peak bone mass rarely occurs before age 25. Therefore, people between the ages 22 and 24 are now included in the previously recommended allowances for the younger, actively growing group aged 19 to 22 years. More vitamin D, thiamine, calcium and phosphorus, and less vitamin K are now recommended for women aged 22 to 24 because of this change in age grouping. Several changes in recommendations for pregnant women have been made since the 1980 edition.

Most industrial countries have their own national recommendations based on research in their populations. Other countries use those set by the World Health Organization (WHO). The dietary standards proposed by WHO may be most appropriate for vegetarians, since they were developed in and for countries in which vegetarian diets predominate.

For example, the American RDA calls for 50 to 60 grams of protein a day for adults (down from a recommendation of 74 grams/day in the 1980s); research that is examined to set this standard is derived from a primarily meat-centered culture. The WHO recommendation is lower—only 44 grams per day—based on cultures where meat protein is far less available. This suggests that far less protein is necessary in a plant-based diet than in a meat-centered one.

Once RDAs have been set, they are then used to develop food groups and dietary plans, and to regulate packaged food content. In the United States, the RDAs are used to create the USRDAs which are required for food labeling nationally. The USRDAs represent the high end of the RDAs, to extend

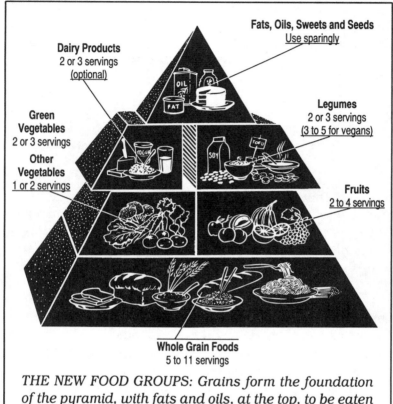

Fats, Oils, Sweets and Seeds
Use sparingly

Dairy Products
2 or 3 servings
(optional)

Legumes
2 or 3 servings
(3 to 5 for vegans)

Green
Vegetables
2 or 3 servings

Other
Vegetables
1 or 2 servings

Fruits
2 to 4 servings

Whole Grain Foods
5 to 11 servings

THE NEW FOOD GROUPS: Grains form the foundation of the pyramid, with fats and oils, at the top, to be eaten only sparingly. Note that dairy products are included as an optional component in this vegetarian diet.

the margin of safety to cover most people under most circumstances.

The "Four Basic Food Groups" that many of us were raised to espouse were developed by the U.S. Department of Agriculture (USDA) in 1956. At that time, there were only eight RDAs, because sufficient information was only available on eight nutrients. The 1990 RDA covers 19 nutrients, plus an additional SADDI (safe and adequate daily dietary intakes) of seven other nutrients.

Creating New Food Groups

On April 8, 1991, the Physicians Committee for Responsible Medicine (PCRM, PO Box 6322, Washington DC 20015) made a proposal to the USDA. The proposal recommended that the USDA adopt a change in the 1956 Four Basic Food Groups to give a more realistic picture of what foods are necessary in a healthy diet. Foods that are now known to be unessential, such as meat products and nuts, are included only as *optional* foods. Research now indicates that, besides being unnecessary, these optional foods may pose a health risk. For example, meats and high fat foods are more likely to contribute to the development of chronic heart disease.

In the new food plan, plants become the center of the diet, quite a change from the USDA's original view. The purpose of the PCRM recommendations was both to decrease risk of heart disease, diabetes and other nutritionally related diseases, and to increase the protective influences of a healthy plant-based diet. As Neal Barnard, the PCRM president, pointed out, it was very possible for people to eat a healthy diet while excluding two of the old food groups completely: meats and dairy products. The two excluded food groups may in fact be detrimental to health, Barnard said, having the highest links with nutritionally related diseases when they are added to the diet.

Taking into consideration the information from the PCRM, the USDA *almost* presented a new food group plan to the public in May, 1991. Fats, oils and sweets were to be used only sparingly, and meat and dairy foods are no longer separate food groups.

Before the revised food grouping was officially published, *The Washington Post* ran a story about it. Meat and dairy groups were threatened by the new design, which minimized the importance of animal products and increased the recommended proportions of grains, vegetables and fruits in the diet. If the U.S. population were ever to switch *en masse* to a plant-centered diet, the meat and dairy industries would suffer a drastic economic loss. The industries attacked the plan by charging that it ranked food into good/bad categories. After heavy pressure, particularly from the National Cattlemen's Association, the proposal was withdrawn for further consideration for over a year, until it was finally released in its pyramid form.

Other Dietary Plans

Since RDAs are primarily a listing of individual nutrient requirements, the development of food recommendations and dietary plans make these requirements practical. An examination of food plans that are developed by various groups and individuals reveals differences that may reflect personal taste preferences rather than nutritional needs. Vegetarian research often cites proposed pregnancy diet plans, but they are not readily available. They are certainly not made a part of most medical reference books on pregnancy; instead, they are subsumed under the omnivore diet, still built around the Four Basic Food Groups of 1956.

The Food Guide Pyramid (USDA 1992)
Daily Recommendations

• Fats, oils, sweets	Not a food group, use sparingly.
• Milk, cheese, yogurt	2-3 servings
• Legumes, meats, dairy	2-3 servings
• Vegetables	3-5 servings
• Fruits	2-4 servings
• Bread, cereal, pasta, rice	6-11 servings

PCRM Food Groups
Daily Recommendations

• Whole grains	5+ servings
• Vegetables	3+ servings
• Legumes	2-3 servings
• Fruits	3+ servings

Michael Klaper's "Vegan Six" Food Groups
Daily Recommendations

Michael Klaper is the author of *Pregnancy, Children and the Vegan Diet.*

• Whole grains and vegetables	2-4 servings, 1 serving = 4 ounces
• Legumes	1-2 servings, 1 serving = 4 ounces
• Green and yellow vegetables	1-3 servings, 1 serving = 4 ounces
• Nuts and seeds	1-3 servings, 1 serving = 1 ounce
• Fruits	3-6 servings, 1 serving = 1 piece

• Vitamin/mineral foods, at least three times a week: 1 serving sea vegetables, 1 serving B_{12} source

Laurel's Kitchen
Daily Recommendations

This is a classic vegetarian handbook and cookbook, first published in 1976 by Laurel Robertson, Carol Flinders and Bronwen Godfrey.

• 60 percent protein from grains
• 35 percent protein from legumes
• 5 percent protein from green leafy vegetables.

These dietary recommendations include more grain and legumes than other vegetarian and vegan food guides. However, the food guide based on *Laurel's Kitchen* is the only dietary plan that Patricia Mutch, reporting in *The American Journal of Clinical Nutrition* (1967), found to meet, or even approach the RDA in energy requirements for pregnant women.

S. Chaij-Rhys
Daily Recommendations

A food guide developed specifically for vegan adults by S. Chaij-Rhys in the late 1970s, was presented by the Seventh-Day Adventist church to its congregations in 1980. Recommendations for the pregnant vegan woman were:

- 2 servings nuts/seeds/protein-rich legumes
- 3 servings milk or meat analogs (such as texturized vegetable protein, TVP)
- 4 servings vegetables
- 5 servings fruits
- 6 servings grains, cereals and breads

This might be called the 2-3-4-5-6 plan. Before publication, the Chaij plan was modified by Seventh-Day Adventist Ethel Martin, who reduced the fruit serving.

Adele Davis
Daily Recommendations

Adele Davis developed a detailed dietary plan for pregnancy in her book, *Let's Have Healthy Children*, but her diet stresses animal foods (especially liver) and high nutrient intake, both of which have controversial aspects.

As you can see in the chart below comparing some of Davis's recommendations with the current RDA for those nutrients, her recommendations for "healthier mothers—superior infants" differs from the RDA for pregnant women in several places:

Nutrient	RDA (10th)	Davis	Variance
Protein	60 g	75-90 g	+15-30 g
Calcium	1,200 mg	2,000 mg	+800 mg
Magnesium	300 mg	800 mg	+500 mg
Iodine	.175 mg	3-4 mg	+2.825-3.825 mg
Vitamin A	1,300 μg	25,000 μg	+23,000 μg
Iron	15 mg	12 mg	-3 mg

Notice that only on iron intake does she recommended a lower dosage; the rest are almost "mega-doses" and would require a lot of supplementation to meet. But she does not believe that high iron intake is good—not only does the body absorb less as more is available, but excess iron in the blood can affect liver and tissue functioning. Iron also interferes with vitamin E absorption, an important healing nutrient. For that reason, most doctors recommend that vitamin E supplements be taken 8 to 12 hours after iron supplements, if both are used.

Although Adele Davis does not recommend iron supplements, she does suggest eating fresh liver once a day and desiccated liver with other meals. Since vegetarians will not be doing this, they might require iron supplements to follow Davis's recommendations.

Macrobiotic Pregnancy Diets
Daily Recommendations

In *Macrobiotic Pregnancy and Care of the Newborn,* Michio and Aveline Kushi recommend the standard macrobiotic diet as basic for pregnant women as well, although modifications "to satisfy needs and cravings" should be taken into account. The basic macrobiotic dietary plan includes:

- 50 to 60 percent of whole grain cereals
- 5 percent (1 to 2 cups) of soup
- 20 to 25 percent (about a quarter of each meal) in vegetables (excluding potatoes, spinach, tomatoes, eggplant and avocado, which should be limited or avoided in the diet)
- 5 to 15 percent beans and sea vegetables

The macrobiotic is particular about which foods can be used and which foods should be avoided. A macrobiotic counselor's advice should be sought if you are considering such a diet during your pregnancy.

Of course, no matter what plans are proposed, what you ultimately eat will be your individualized dietary plan. If you have a healthy diet to start with, eating to meet the needs of your naturally increased appetite during pregnancy will probably satisfy almost all of your dietary needs. But if you locate weaknesses in your diet before conception, such as not eating enough fresh vegetables, try to improve this into a good habit. Checking against the New Four Food Groups as proposed by the PCRM may be the simplest way to make sure your diet is varied and complete enough.

Personal Experiences
Bunny Chidester

One of the things that helped me the most during my second (vegan) pregnancy was keeping a daily food chart. I designed it from a list of six vegan food groups in Dr. Klaper's book, *Pregnancy, Children, and the Vegan Diet.* I listed each group, what was in it, and how many servings were suggested a day. Then I made small boxes to check off each serving I ate each day. I made copies of my food chart and would hang one on my kitchen cabinet every day. This gave me a clear view of what areas needed improvement (usually greens and fruits), and where I was doing okay. I enjoyed keeping the chart, and it was a good way for my midwife to see that I was eating well. She was totally supportive of vegetarianism/veganism during pregnancy, which helped me a lot.

Further Information

• "A diet pattern for total vegetarians" by S. Chaij-Rhys, *Adventist Review*, 1980, 157:1014-1015.

• "Development of a culturally appropriate food guide for pregnant Caribbean immigrants in the United States" by Sharon L. Stowers, *Journal of the American Dietetic Association*, March, 1992, Vol. 92, No. 3, 331-336. (Reports that the traditional Four Food Groups are not adequate to meet the needs of pregnant vegetarians or most immigrant ethnic groups of pregnant women.)

• "Food Guides for the Vegetarian" by Patricia B. Mutch, *American Journal of Clinical Nutrition*, 1988, 48:913-919.

• "Food Guide Pyramid Replaces Basic 4 Circle" in *Food Technology*, July 1992, 62-64.

• *Laurel's Kitchen* by Laurel Robertson, *et al.*, Ten Speed Press, Berkeley, CA, 1992.

• *Let's Have Healthy Children* by Adele Davis, New American Library, New York, NY, 1972.

• *Macrobiotic Pregnancy and Care of the Newborn* by Michio and Aveline Kushi, Japan Publications, New York, NY, 1985.

• Physicians Committee for Responsible Medicine, PO Box 6322, Washington DC 20015, (202) 686-2210.

• *Pregnancy, Children and the Vegan Diet* by Michael Klaper, Gentle World Inc, Maui, HI, 1987.

• *The Food Guide Pyramid* by the Human Nutrition Information Service, Home and Garden Bulletin Number 352, available free from U.S. Department of Agriculture, Human Nutrition Information service, 6505 Belcrest Road, Hyattsville, MD 20782.

HEARTBURN

Heartburn, a strong discomfort in the upper stomach/esophagus area of the digestive tract, is experienced by at least 30 percent of women during pregnancy. It is felt most commonly soon after eating, as a burning sensation in the chest and throat area, near the heart, hence the misnomer "heartburn."

Heartburn is common during pregnancy because the stomach area is reduced as the baby grows. Particularly during the final months of pregnancy, the baby pushes upwards against the stomach as well as downwards against the intestines. With a smaller space in the stomach for recently eaten food, a raised level of stomach acids, and a slowed digestive process, your stomach will feel (and actually be) fuller more frequently. Internal pressure causes stomach acids to move up the esophagus, causing a burning sensation in the chest (heart) area.

Recommendations

• Rich, fatty, fried and hot spicy foods are most likely to cause heartburn, so they should be eaten sparingly.

• Small, frequent meals chewed well are the best form of prevention for heartburn.

• When eating, sit up straight, allowing maximum room for the stomach. After eating, take a leisurely walk around to stimulate digestion while maintaining maximum space for your full stomach. Keep your head up.

• If you need to lie down soon after eating, make sure you prop yourself up at a 30° angle to keep stomach acids on a gravitationally downward motion. You may also want to sleep in a semi-upright position if heartburn bothers you at night.

• Don't eat too much before going to bed, to keep the stomach from being too full. Don't eat too little either, as that may produce hunger pains (excess stomach acid without food to digest).

• Don't drink a lot when you eat, but drink enough between meals. This will keep you from getting too full at meals, and will dilute the stomach acids between meals.

• Calcium has been called nature's antacid. It neutralizes stomach acids and generally makes the digestive process more efficient. Don't take commercial antacids which contain ingredients that may be harmful to the fetus.

• Ginger root, anise, fennel seed and slippery elm bark teas are recommended by many herbalists for easing heartburn. Slippery elm throat lozenges have been suggested as a way to neutralize stomach acids. Chewing a natural mint gum has also been found to help soothe heartburn.

• Chewing on small amounts of raw almonds, organic fruit peels (particularly apple peels) and papaya will help problems with indigestion and heartburn.

INFERTILITY

A diagnosis of infertility is commonly applied if conception does not occur after one year of regular intercourse without the use of contraception. Infertility may be caused by a male's sperm not being strong or numerous enough to survive the trip to the egg, or by an egg which is not released or cannot be fertilized. The causes of infertility, both physical and emotional, are numerous but there are several points at which nutrition interacts with an inability to conceive.

In Women

An April 1986 study, reported in *The American Journal of Clinical Nutrition* found that vegetarian women were more likely to have irregular menstrual cycles than non-vegetarian women. This was most likely the result of their lower carbohydrate intake, common especially in vegan diets since plant foods have far less caloric value than any or all meats and meat products. Vegan women are more likely (according to stereotype at least) to be underweight than meat-eating women.

Women who are underweight are less likely to conceive. Underweight women are more likely to miss periods and have fewer periods. Irregular menstrual cycles can make conception more difficult, since ovulation won't be predictable.

If you are planning to get pregnant, check your diet to make sure you include enough carbohydrate foods. If you are getting only minimal calories and your menstrual cycles are irregular, eat extra breads, grains, cereals and soups. If you have not already done so, it might be worthwhile to read up on the signs of ovulation, such as increased mucus, to be sure to know when you are most likely to conceive. (See *Further Information*, below)

The June 22, 1991 issue of *Lancet*, a weekly scientific chronicle, reported that conception may be prevented in women with both low iron and vitamin C levels. Supplementation of these two nutrients increased the chances of pregnancy "significantly" (7⅓ times).

An earlier issue of *Lancet* (May 11, 1991) reported that caffeinated soft drinks may impair a woman's fertility, whereas teas were *not* associated with a lower fertility. Black teas and coffees high in caffeine may reduce fertility, but not as much as soft drinks do.

Several reports in the news have indicated that well-off white women are more likely to encounter infertility than others. This is probably the result of waiting until later in life to have children; a woman in her 20s is more fertile than a woman in her 40s, given similar diets. Irregular menstrual cycles, stress and changing hormonal balances due to aging can contribute to infertility in older women.

Several herbal tea preparations have been recommended as fertility promoters among women. These teas use herbs such as red raspberry leaves, dong quai root, red clover leaves and nettle leaves, most of which are available through a health foods store or natural foods mail order businesses. The plants help to regularize the hormonal system and tone the uterus, thus increasing the chances of ovulation and successful egg implantation. In addition, extra vitamins A and E, calcium and magnesium, particularly in food form, may be helpful in encouraging fertility. (See "Supplementation")

In Men

Dr. John MacLeod of the Cornell University Medical School was one of the first researchers to note that sperm counts have been decreasing in males, in particular, males in the United States. Average sperm count declined from about 90 million/count in the 1920s to about 65 million/count in 1975 (a "count" is a milliliter of sperm), a plummeting drop of 25 million! (See "Conception")

Both sperm and eggs are vulnerable to environmental toxins. A lowered sperm count can be caused by exposure to toxins, a deficiency of manganese or zinc, or a deficiency in the diet of almost any of the vitamins. Smoking, excessive alcohol and insufficient exercise also contribute to lowered fertility in men.

Since the cause of infertility is at least partly nutritional, it may be possible to provide a remedy. For example, an experimentally induced zinc deficit in a group of men significantly reduced their sperm count. A zinc supplement was then added to their diet and regular sperm levels were restored after 6 to 12 months.

This does not indicate that Adele Davis's recommendation that zinc supplements of 250 mg/day for prospective fathers is appropriate for all prospective parents—not at all! The National Research Council reviewed several studies on excessive intake of zinc. Their conclusion was that doses of more than 15 mg/day over a long period of time were not recommended without adequate supervision. Doses of 300 mg/day reduced the effectiveness of the immune system in various tests done by R.K. Chandra in 1984.

However, if the father's zinc level is too low, as determined by someone with medical knowledge of testing for zinc levels in the body, specific zinc supplementation doses may be prescribed for the male. The normal zinc level in semen is 90 to 250 μg/ml. Since taking zinc supplements without accurate testing is risky self-medicating, a far better approach is to eat plenty of foods rich in zinc.

In June 1992, *Vegetarian Times* reported that, according to a study in the *Proceedings of the National Academy of Sciences*, men should have at least 250 mg of vitamin C each day to avoid an increased risk of fathering children with genetic defects, leukemia and lymphoma.

Deficiencies in manganese (an essential trace mineral) and several other vitamins are also implicated in male infertility. The following RDAs are for men between the ages of 15 and 50 and should be met by men planning to be fathers.

Zinc: 15 mg/day (Eat more sunflower seeds, mushrooms, brewer's yeast, soybeans.)

Manganese: 2.0-5.0 mg/day (Eat more whole grains, green leafy vegetables, legumes, nuts, pineapples.)

Vitamin A: 1,000 μg RE (Retinol Equivalent) = 1 μg retinol or 6 μg beta-carotene (Eat more yellow fruits/vegetables, dark green fruits/vegetables.)

Vitamin E: 10 μg sigma-TE (Tocopherol Equivalent) = 10 mg d-sigma tocopherol (Use more cold-pressed oils in cooking and salads, eat more wheat germ, molasses, sweet potatoes, leafy vegetables.)

Pantothenic Acid: 4 to 7 mg/day (Eat more brewer's yeast, wheat germ, legumes, whole grains.)

Vitamin B_{12}: 2.0 μg/day (You must take a supplement if you are a vegan who eats no dairy or eggs.)

The macrobiotic approach to infertility suggests that dishes strongly seasoned with sea salt, miso or tamari should be added to the diet more frequently to increase the yang energy. Yin foods such as fruits, salads and nuts should be minimized for several months during the period a couple is trying to conceive.

Further Information
• "Tea and Fertility" by A.J. Wilcox and C.R. Weinherg, *Lancet*, May 11, 1991.
• *What You Can Do About Infertility*, by Pamela Patrick Novotny, Dell Publishing, New York, NY, 1991. (Lots of technical information.)
• *Wise Woman Herbal for the Childbearing Year* by Susun S. Weed, Ash Tree Publishing, Woodstock, NY 1986. (For specifics on herbal teas and much more.)

Personal Experiences
Lynn Semega
Many of my friends who were approaching 40 were having fertility problems. Some had been trying for years to conceive. I had one unprotected night with my boyfriend and ended up pregnant. I believe that my good health, via a vegetarian diet, kept my body young and able to conceive easily.

INSOMNIA

Many women report changes in their sleeping patterns as pregnancy progresses. This is a natural change as your body gets ready to feed the newborn on a 24-hour schedule.

You may need to alter your regular sleeping positions in order to be comfortable in the later months of pregnancy. These changes may make your sleep less restful unless you can introduce alternate positions that are just as relaxing. Extra pillows can make lying on your side more comfortable. It will be easier on your back if you sleep on your side after the fifth month.

Because your stomach has less room in later pregnancy, lying completely flat on your back (particularly if you are used to sleeping with a pillow) will increase the feeling of heartburn. To ease that, use an extra pillow as a prop for your upper back and head.

Vigorous exercise, caffeine and large, heavy or spicy meals too close to bedtime can make getting to sleep difficult and sleep itself restless. If you drink milk, drink a little before bed. It contains tryptophan, which will relax you. Or, if you don't drink milk, try a warm, gentle tea like chamomile for the same effect.

LOW ENERGY

Low energy is commonly experienced by women in the first trimester of pregnancy. In contrast, most women seem to feel very healthy and energetic during the second trimester. During the final three months, the baby has grown so much that almost everyone is slowed down by the extra weight.

These energy levels reflect the metabolic changes of pregnancy and are designed by nature to help the mother know what is best for a developing fetus. Initial fatigue is caused by a major increase in progesterone which slows down the digestive system for more efficient nutrient use. All the muscles are relaxed as the skeletal structure adjusts to carry and give birth to a baby. The internal changes of early pregnancy are often unnoticeable externally, but the start of a new life requires a tremendous energy output, leaving less available for normal functioning.

By the second trimester, appetite has increased to match the additional energy needed for the developing fetus, and most women find they feel healthiest and most active during this time.

By the third trimester, energy is primarily used to increase the baby's weight and to help the mother constantly carry the accumulated 25 to 30 extra pounds most women gain over this nine-month period. (See "Weight Gain")

Low energy can also result from a dietary imbalance with too many simple sugars and empty calories and too few complex sugars and healthy carbohydrates. Caffeine may produce an immediate increase in energy, but it takes more than it gives and, consumed in too great a quantity, will ultimately sap essential energy necessary for healthy fetal development. (See "Toxins") Sweets do the same thing, providing an initial rush of extra energy that ends up leaving you worn out and depleted in B and C vitamins, with lower blood sugar than when you started.

Low energy might discourage exercise but, frequently, too little activity contributes to a greater feeling of exhaustion. Without the overall stimulation of physical activity, digestion is less efficient and important nutrients are more likely to be excreted before they are properly assimilated.

Although meat-eaters may contend that a lack of meat in the diet can cause fatigue, research shows no decrease in the physical stamina of new vegetarians. In fact, subjectively, the new vegetarians reported feeling more energetic. The fats in meat make it difficult and slow to digest, so it makes sense that those eating meat had to spend more energy on digestion and had less to spare for other activities, unlike the vegetarians.

Recommendations

• Get enough exercise; at minimum, a half hour of walking a day. Gentle exercise keeps oxygen readily available and the body stimulated.

• Even if you don't do yoga, take a little time out to try deep, slow breathing in a supine or standing position. This will increase blood flow and oxygen throughout the body.

• Eat natural energy-producing foods: bananas, carrots, dates, figs, peas, spinach and strawberries are all considered "energy foods." Avoid processed foods, especially in excess.

• Dairy products, particularly milk, contain tryptophan, a natural sedative. This might be helpful if you need to rest, but may add to fatigue if you have started to drink more milk during pregnancy, on a doctor's advice. (See "Milk and Dairy Products" for alternatives to milk during pregnancy.)

• Peppermint and spearmint teas are known to renew a sense of energy. Iced mint tea in the summer can help cut through immobilizing summer heat.

• Listen to your body when it needs to rest.

• Be sure you have sufficient iron. Although it is normal to feel fatigue at times during pregnancy, it can also be a symptom of an iron deficiency. (See "Anemia" and "Understanding Nutrients: Iron") Eating iron-rich foods, such as dark dried fruits, provides extra iron, other nutrients and natural energy.

MACROBIOTIC PREGNANCY

At its core, macrobiotics rests on a philosophy of balance. This includes the belief that ideal balance within the human body is facilitated by diet. It is this notion which has caused a great deal of confusion about the healthiness of a macrobiotic diet. Sometimes, a vegetarian diet may be accepted for a pregnant woman while a macrobiotic one will not.

Scientific research has only compounded this confusion, with early studies of vegetarianism reporting on children raised in macrobiotic households where principles of good nutrition were overrun by ignorance and good intent. People who fear vegetarian pregnancies in their friends and loved ones are often victims of the spread of such cultural misinformation.

Macrobiotic diets and vegetarian diets may be the same in content—or they may not. Vegetarians, by definition, do not eat meat. Macrobiotics—by definition—strive to achieve a balance within their diet. Macrobiotic diets frequently exclude meat because a vegetarian diet is healthier for the body, providing a preferable balance within, regardless of ethical values.

Michio and Aveline Kushi, students of George Ohsawa, who introduced macrobiotics to the Western world, are primary resources for macrobiotic pregnant women. Like most books on pregnancy, their book, *Macrobiotic Pregnancy and the Care of the Newborn*, is filled with basic nutritional and health information that is unchanged by cultural setting. However, it also contains particular warnings about animal foods during pregnancy.

For example, they believe that animal foods will weaken the egg. Animal fats and proteins in the sperm may strengthen the sperm, but they may also cause blockage in the tubes which carry sperm from the testes to the penis. In women, animal foods are believed to contribute to infertility. When pregnant women crave animal foods (meats and milks), the Kushis recommend rich bean foods such as tempeh, seitan, tofu and natto, root vegetables and miso condiments as an alternative balance.

One questionable comment the Kushis make is that morning sickness indicates an imbalance in the system. Current research seems to show that, in fact, this very common experience exists for the innately healthy purpose of protecting and defining the mother's food intake. (See "Nausea")

A 1991 contributor to *Macrobiotics Today* wrote to suggest that macrobiotic diets may need to include more salt, miso and shoyu than other diets, for proper digestion of grains and vegetables. While she did not refer specifically to the needs of pregnancy, this is an important point—not only for macrobiotics, but for all who shun the use of salt in their diets. During pregnancy, digestion is normally more sluggish, and proper sodium intake is essential to avoid slowing the process even more. (See "Salt," "Digestion" and "Constipation")

In their discussion of balance in the body during pregnancy, the Kushis consistently emphasize the importance of women listening to their own body signals, and trusting that information. While they give many specific macrobiotic recipes, the Kushis also deeply respect the wisdom and needs transmitted by the pregnant woman's body. They suggest fish foods frequently, but always offer alternative vegetable choices.

Most research regarding macrobiotics focuses on possible deficiencies of calcium, vitamin D and iron, as well as vitamin B_{12} if the diet is also vegan. These nutrients are of concern to all pregnant women, no matter their dietary preference. Children born to macrobiotic and vegan women have registered lower weight and length measurements at birth than other children, but this is primarily a result of lower carbohydrate intake rather than an innate drawback of the diet. Since larger babies have a lower incidence of problems both at birth and in the first few years of life, it is wise to let the natural increase in your appetite during pregnancy be an internal guide to achieving balance within. In other words, eat plenty of healthy complex carbohydrates for a healthier child. (See "Weight Gain" and "Understanding Nutrients: Carbohydrates, Calcium, Vitamin D, Vitamin B_{12}")

Further Information
* *Macrobiotic Pregnancy* by Alice Feinberg, George Ohsawa Macrobiotic Foundation, Los Angeles, CA, 1973.
* *Macrobiotic Pregnancy and Care of the Newborn, Revised Edition* by Michio and Aveline Kushi, Japan Publications, New York, NY, 1985.
* "Salt Fears Unfounded," letter by Rachel Albert, *Macrobiotics Today*, Sept-Oct 1991, p.4.

Personal Experiences

Nancy Rankin

I had been a macrobiotic cooking teacher for six years prior to motherhood. Six weeks into pregnancy, all my pre-conceived ideas went out the window. I became extremely nauseous, and could no more conceive of eating brown rice and miso soup, then stand in my kitchen to prepare it. For the first half of my pregnancy I subsisted on endless bowls of cereal, soymilk and fruit. This was not the diet I had imagined I would consume to nourish my baby. I weighed the chatter in my head with my body's attraction to foods that suited my changing nutritional needs. Sometimes yogurt tasted and felt appropriate. Gradually my tastes widened and whole grains, beans, land and sea vegetables, nuts and seeds once again graced my plate in increasing amounts. I had redefined my macrobiotic label to reflect the art of making balance.

Deborah McGrath

In my third pregnancy, I became interested in macrobiotics. I had read a lot about it, and thought that the philosophy behind it made sense. I found many cookbooks and wonderful recipes to try. Some ingredients and foods were not always easy to obtain at the health food store or a local Oriental market, but I found an excellent mail order company to round out my shopping needs.

My doctor was concerned about my macrobiotic diet because it doesn't use soy milk or cheese. I did find a wonderful tea which is a staple of the macrobiotic diet, called bancha. It is loaded with calcium, and supplies more calcium than dairy products, without the fat. I loved the bancha tea, and many other basic macrobiotic foods, such as miso soup. This pregnancy and labor was the easiest of all three, and I believe that nutrition played a major role.

Paula Borenstein

I attended Bradley childbirth class and, at first, the instructor was skeptical that I could fulfill my protein and calcium requirements on a macrobiotic diet. I kept faithful track of what I ate as part of the class, and added up my calcium and protein intake. I was getting at least enough, and sometimes a little extra. She never doubted my diet after that and I brought in recipes and samples of my cooking for others to try.

MEAT AND MEAT HAZARDS

It may seem strange to have information about meat and meat hazards presented to a vegetarian audience. However, chances are you will still be pressured about not eating meat while you are pregnant, so this section is mostly for "vegetarian self-defense" (the title of a 1979 book by Richard Bargen). Pregnant or not, good reasons to avoid meat abound, and having this information available may be useful when a doctor or well-meaning friends try to tell you how important and healthy it is to eat meat, *especially* during pregnancy.

Foods of animal origin are a tremendous source of pesticide residues. The fats in animal foods are particularly well adapted to permanent storage of such chemicals—until they are digested by a human. The Environmental Protection Agency itself has pointed this out, as well as the Food and Drug Administration. But meat-eating is so central to our culture that the logical steps of either excluding animal foods from the diet or preventing the animals' exposure to pesticides and hormones is ignored.

Sick animals are treated with large amounts of antibiotics and sulfa drugs. Even though the entire animal may not be salvageable for food, parts are routinely saved, despite the high levels of drugs they contain. Herbicides and pesticides are used on crops that are raised to feed animals. The chemical toxins are passed along the food chain, ending up in fresh and frozen meats and meat products.

Hormones to increase rate and size of growth (such as steroids) are regularly added to animal feed and end up in the human diet when meat is eaten. In 1987, it was reported that about 99 percent of all commercially raised cattle were treated with growth hormones. Synovex is one of the more common. It is implanted into the ears of animals and produces great increases in weight gain.

Animals are fed pesticide "protected" foods year after year, and the toxins accumulate. They can't be washed off, as chemicals can from many plant foods, and they are rarely broken down within the animals, even over a period of time. Jeremy Rifkin's important book, *Beyond Beef*, offers but one of the many descriptions of the horrors of the meat industry, whose main goal has always been to increase the quantity of meat produced, bypassing legal restrictions all too frequently.

Red meats are bad for our health even if they are produced on organic farms. The overload of protein, the fat and the cholesterol content of red meats is well-documented as a risky addition to the diet. The new food groups presented by the U.S. Department of Agriculture present meats as a food to limit in the diet. (See "Food Groups, Dietary Plans and RDAs") This is a stark change from the old "Four Food Groups" (still adhered to by many nutritionists!) which have meat as one of the four, and milk/dairy as another.

The use of pesticides and hormones in animal foods is fairly recent. As more and more toxins are stored in animals, levels of contamination are becoming increasingly dangerous. Already, U.S. national awareness of the dangers in meat production industries is growing and by the end of the century, the wider population may consider meats as dangerous as cigarettes and drugs to fetal and maternal health.

Fish is one of the last meat foods given up by vegetarians, and fish dishes are sometimes included in vegetarian cookbooks. Fish, however, reflect the heavy environmental damage and chemical waste pollution of the major bodies of water inside the United States. Swordfish, marlin and bluefish are particularly dangerous, and any fish from the Great Lakes and the Hudson River should be completely avoided during pregnancy (and in general). Freshwater carp, wild catfish, lake trout, mackerel, striped bass and whitefish are likely to contain high levels of PCBs and should not be eaten either.

Milk, dairy and eggs are likely to be high in toxins because they are fatty foods. (See "Milk and Dairy Products" and "Eggs") Organically raised animals still contain high levels of fat and cholesterol. Meat is hard to digest because of its concentrated fat and protein and will make the slowed digestion process of pregnancy very sluggish. (See "Digestion") Additionally, meat that moves through the body slowly will tend to rot and putrefy within the body. The toxins from this process are not healthy for the baby or the mother.

Avoiding meat during pregnancy is one of the best actions you can take to assure your baby a healthy early life. Many pregnant women feel a revulsion for meat during pregnancy even when no such feeling occurred before. (See "Cravings and Aversions") This may be a natural mechanism to protect the fetus.

Further Information
(Especially recommended to those who think meat is good for you; vegetarians may find many of the descriptions of the meat industry upsetting and unnecessary to read during pregnancy)

• *Animals and Society: The Humanity of Animal Rights*, by Keith Tester, Routledge Chapman Hall, New York, NY, 1991.

• *Animal Factories*, by Jim Mason and Peter Singer, Harmony/Crown, New York, NY, 1990.

• *Beyond Beef: the Rise and Fall of the Cattle Culture*, by Jeremy Rifkin, Dutton, New York, NY, 1992.

• *Diet for a Small Planet, Revised Edition*, by Frances Moore Lappé, Ballantine Books, New York, NY, 1990.

• Physicians Committee for Responsible Medicine, PO Box 6322, Washington D.C. 20015 (An organization that is "working to achieve better health for people through humane treatment of animals").

• *Safe Food: Eating Wisely in a Risky World*, by Michael F. Jacobson, *et al.*, Living Planet Press, Venice, CA, 1991; chapters 3 (Milk and Cheese), 4 (Meat, Poultry and Eggs), and 5 (Fish and Shellfish).

• *Vegetarian's Self-defense Manual*, by Richard Bargen, Theosophical Publishing House, Wheaton, IL, 1979.

MILK AND DAIRY PRODUCTS

Is drinking milk necessary during pregnancy? Many doctors, family and friends may say so, but it is not true. Drinking milk is one way of getting calcium and protein, but certainly not the only way. In September, 1992, the Physicians Committee for Responsible Medicine held a news conference to report that milk was not the ideal protein nor should it be a primary protein, as had originally been thought. The PCRM, a non-profit group of doctors, including child care expert Dr. Benjamin Spock, was primarily concerned about the problems of giving milk, particularly whole milk, to children because of the high percentage of fat, the probable connection to juvenile diabetes, colic, allergies and digestive problems. However, the major point of the news conference was to increase nutritional awareness and consumption of healthier forms of calcium, such as broccoli, leafy vegetables, tahini and tofu made with calcium sulfate.

The most recent RDA standards for calcium intake (1989) were put at 1,200 mg/day for pregnant adults (higher for pregnant teenagers). This is about 300 mg/day more than recommended for a non-pregnant female. Most people absorb only 20 to 30 percent of their calcium intake, or about 240 mg/day. During pregnancy, women increase their efficiency in calcium use, absorbing a higher percentage. This increase in efficiency also occurs when calcium intake comes from plant sources rather than animal sources (animal fat may impede the process of calcium absorption).

The amount of protein in the diet also affects the efficiency of calcium absorption. The greater the amount of protein eaten, the lower the rate of calcium use will be. Milk, a form of calcium clothed in animal fats and protein, is not a very effective way to get either calcium or protein into the mother's body, even though it is quite high in both. In a study of Swedish vegans, blood levels of calcium were the same as in omnivore women, despite almost half the calcium intake.

If you drink milk, or were brought up as I was, to believe that three glasses of milk were essential to good health, this information may come as a surprise. It may not change your mind about drinking milk, but it should make you realize that it is not necessary to drink milk to obtain sufficient calcium or protein, even if you are pregnant.

Some women develop an aversion to milk during pregnancy. (See "Cravings and Aversions") Others develop a craving for it. Thoughts of cheese, yogurt and other dairy products may produce binge attacks or become distasteful; experiences vary. For many vegetarians, since milk can be obtained from a cow or goat without harming the animal, drinking milk may not be an issue. Others object to any animal foods in the diet, entirely for health reasons. The one fact to remember through all the emotional debate is that you do not need to include milk, dairy or eggs in your diet during pregnancy or during any other stage of life.

However, if you don't get calcium and protein from milk, it is essential to get it elsewhere, especially during pregnancy. (See "Understanding Nutrients: Calcium and Protein") A diet based on leafy green vegetables and legumes will provide sufficient calcium, even taking into account the greater calcium absorption rate found in vegans. As Gill Langley reports in a 1988 survey of research on vegans, no finding of calcium deficiency in adult vegans has turned up.

Tofu processed with calcium sulfate will have 250 to 765 mg of calcium per 4 ounces. If the tofu is made with nigari (magnesium chloride), it will be lower in calcium content, but still a major calcium source to include in your diet. A cup of cooked collard greens has over 350 mg and spinach and turnip greens also provide about the same amount per cup. If you are used to eating these greens in your diet, you are probably getting sufficient calcium. Many legumes such as pinto beans, black beans and soybeans also have at least 100 mg of calcium per one-half cup of cooked beans.

Beans simultaneously provide protein and calcium, while greens provide minerals and vitamins along with calcium. Drinking milk does not measure up as a substitute for a good vegan diet. If milk and dairy products are a staple of your diet, be sure to enrich it with plenty of plant foods for the healthiest pregnancy.

Pasteurized milk and cheeses are naturally filled with animal fats and are therefore carry all the pesticides, growth hormones and other chemical residues the animals may have picked up. Recently it was reported that vitamin D is routinely added to milk "above and beyond" the legal requirements, and too much vitamin D can be toxic. (See "Nutrients: Vitamin D") Most cheese products are made with rennet, an enzyme from the stomach of cattle or pigs. Such cheeses cannot be called vegetarian.

A microbial enzyme, used by health food companies such as Walnut Acres, is neither animal or vegetable. Soy cheeses can be made with or without casein, a milk protein, but do not contain rennet; those without casein are usually different in texture than other cheeses and do not melt as well.

However, for vegans especially, this kind of cheese is a great way to get calcium and protein in the diet.

Some green vegetables, particularly spinach and chard, contain oxalic acid, which inhibits the absorption of calcium. There has been some evidence that long-term vegans adjust to plant greens as a source of calcium by developing the digestive ability to override calcium inhibitors.

Rice, more than any other grain, contains a substance that neutralizes oxalic acid. If rice is eaten in the same meal with spinach or chard, the calcium in the greens becomes available once again. Remember, Popeye may have had rice pudding for dessert!

Other greens, like kale, mustard greens, and collards, are very low in oxalates and are excellent sources of calcium. To assure sufficient calcium in your diet without milk, eat a variety of green vegetables, favoring spinach and chard with rice dishes and other greens with other grains. Beans, nut milks, seed butters (such as tahini), and calcium-fortified soy milk are also good sources of calcium and should be incorporated into a vegan diet (especially) on a daily basis.

Recommendations

• Keep milk and dairy intake to a minimum but be sure to eat lots of other calcium-rich foods (See "Nutrients: Calcium") which provide additional vitamins and minerals without fats and possible contamination by pesticides, insecticides or hormones.

• Eat rice in meals with spinach and chard to block the calcium-binding effects of oxalic acid found in those foods.

• Buy fresh leafy vegetables—organically grown, if possible.

• Make sure that tofu you buy has been made with calcium sulfate (it should say on the label; with bulk tofu at a health foods store, you may have to ask the person who buys it for the store).

Further Information

- "Calcium utilization: effect of varying level and source of dietary protein" by Michael B. Zemel, *American Journal of Clinical Nutrition*, 1988; 48:880-883.
- "Cow's Milk and Children: a new no-no?" by Marian Burros, *The New York Times*, September 30, 1992.
- *Dairy-free Cookbook*, by Jane Zukin, Prima Publishing, Rocklin, CA, 1991.
- "Milk's nutritional value questioned," Associated Press news item, *The Ithaca Journal*, September 29, 1992.
- *Safe Food: Eating Wisely in a Risky World*, by Michael F. Jacobson *et al.*, Living Planet Press, Venice, CA, 1991 (particularly Chapter 3, Milk and Cheese).
- *Simply Vegan: Quick Vegetarian Meals*, by Debra Wasserman, Vegetarian Resource Group, Baltimore, MD, 1991.
- *The Book of Tofu*, by William Shurtleff and Akiko Aoyagi, Ballantine Books, New York, NY, 1979.
- "The Effect of Dairy Products on Iron Availability," by Lauren S. Jackson and Ken Lee in *Critical Views in Food Science and Nutrition*, 1992, 31 (4):259-270.
- *The Tofu Book*, by John Paino and Lisa Messinger, Avery Publications, New York, NY, 1991.
- *Transition to Vegetarianism* by Rudolph Ballentine, Himalayan International Institute, Honesdale, PA, 1987.
- *Vegan Nutrition: A Survey of Research* by Gill Langley, Vegan Society, East Sussex, England, 1988.

Personal Experiences
Monica Leal

I was concerned about calcium and simply did not have the knowledge of how to obtain enough calcium on a vegan diet while pregnant. I decided to err on the side of excess and drank huge amounts of raw certified goat's milk throughout the pregnancy. Big mistake! Although goat's milk is more assimilable and less mucus-producing than pasteurized cow's milk, it is extremely high in fat. I knew this at the time but figured I wouldn't have any trouble losing the weight later.

Wrong! I gained 20 pounds more than I was supposed to and three years later still have not taken it off. Keep in mind that I exercised regularly (five times a week) during my pregnancy and have continued to do so since. I never touch ice cream, butter, sodas or any of those other dietary "evils." I believe goat's milk was the culprit and now I stay away from all milk.

Sharon Outten
Many of our new Army friends were also expecting babies. Most of them felt that we were a little nutty to be vegetarian, but we never preached to them. As the months passed, they began to notice the differences between their pregnancies and mine, and that's when they began to ask a lot of questions.

They were surprised that I didn't have leg cramps since I drank almost no milk and ate little of other dairy products. I explained that I drank freshly made carrot juice almost daily during the last trimester, much as they drank milk daily. They were surprised to learn how much calcium carrots and other vegetables contain. My boss and co-workers were truly amazed at my endurance and cheerfulness. I worked from my third month until two weeks before our baby was born. During that time I won three awards for service and friendliness to customers.

NAUSEA/MORNING SICKNESS

Nausea, "a feeling of sickness in the stomach with an impulse to vomit" *(Webster's New World Dictionary, Third College Edition)* is very common during pregnancy, particularly in the first trimester, and particularly first thing in the morning, hence the pregnancy-specific category of "morning sickness." At least 70 percent of pregnant women experience this nausea.

Nausea is of course an unpleasant problem, but it has been positively linked with healthy births! Although the mechanisms involved are not clearly understood, it appears that early pregnancy nausea might be a natural protective device, protecting a woman from eating many normal foods, and almost forcing her to take extra-special care of herself at a time when the fetus needs a healthy and stable environment.

Research on this subject has been done most recently and definitively by Dr. Margie Profet, a biologist at the University of California, Berkeley. In Profet's view, morning sickness is a natural mechanism to help pregnant women temporarily avoid foods that are likely to contain natural toxins, including many vegetables, spices and fruits which have native defense chemicals to help fend off insect pests. The result is that women with morning sickness will tend to seek out a bland, low-toxin diet of breads and cereals, which eases the nausea.

The placenta is not fully formed until the third month of pregnancy; its tissues are thicker and less permeable until that time. Thus the developing fetus receives extra protection in its most vunerable first months. It is very important for the immediate fetal environment to be stable during this delicate time and the placenta acts as a strong buffer between the mother's nutrition and the developing child.

However, it may be that nausea during the first trimester helps set the course for a healthier diet and lifestyle during the next two trimesters, in effect cleansing the mother's body of toxins during the safest time for the developing fetus. Women who experience morning sickness have a higher incidence of healthy births than women who do not. Of course, extreme nausea can very well indicate an imbalance in the body and is likely not healthy, in contrast to a limited queasiness with which some food can be kept down.

Not all women experience nausea during pregnancy, and the severity differs from person to person. Nausea may occur not only in the morning, nor only during the first trimester. Pregnancy can be particularly difficult for women who have little relief from nausea for an extended period, in some cases the whole length of their pregnancy. If you are in this situation, talk to your doctor about the possibility of prescribing a vitamin B_6 supplement (25 mg/day), which has frequently helped to alleviate the worst symptoms. Be sure to monitor your diet to make sure it's healthy, even if the quantities you're eating are reduced because of the nausea.

Comfort and support from family and doctors becomes crucial when the physical experience of pregnancy is less than pleasant due to extended morning sickness. Often tension and stress can make digestion more difficult; a relaxed person will absorb nutrients more efficiently (something the pregnant body knows as it sends out progesterone to slow the muscle action of the digestive system).

Nausea may be triggered by particular odors or by taste. (See "Sensory Changes") In fact, many women find meat unappealing during their pregnancy even if they were not vegetarians before. It is not surprising that meats, so likely to contain toxins (see Meat and Meat Hazards), would be something women might be naturally inclined to avoid during the important early period of pregnancy.

Morning sickness may also be related to the raised estrogen levels of pregnancy, lowered blood sugar in the morning, and increased acids in the stomach, all of which exist to balance the natural slowing of the digestion during pregnancy. (See "Constipation")

Besides the obvious unpleasantness, nausea is of concern because it lowers a mother's nutritional intake—feeling sick, she just eats less. Don't feel pressured to eat a lot if you are not hungry, but if your total intake is minimal, this is an important time to eat only healthy foods.

In some women, nausea, loss of appetite and/or an inability to keep food down during the first weeks may be the indication of a nutritional imbalance. A generally poor diet immediately prior to pregnancy and in the early weeks will increase nausea. Many of these early morning sickness signs may also be symptoms of a vitamin B_6 deficiency; some evidence shows that a B_6 supplement can ease the unpleasant symptoms.

The RDA for vitamin B_6 is 2.2 mg per day. Adele Davis recommended taking 10 mg of vitamin B_6 daily for a month or two before pregnancy, or 250 mg daily if nausea during pregnancy has already started. The first recommendations of B_6 for this purpose grew out of three separate experiments during the 1940s, in which dosages from 5 to 100 mg/day were added as a supplement to women's diets to ease nausea and vomiting. Proper control groups were not in place during these experiments, however, and some later studies suggest that a placebo effect in these circumstances probably works as well to reduce symptoms—in other words, if you think a little extra B_6 will help you, it probably will.

The Vitamin B_6 complex is found in:

avocados	1 avocado	=.84 mg
bananas	1 banana	=.76 mg
nutritional yeast	1 oz	=.56 mg
wheat germ (toasted)	1/2 cup	=.55 mg
cantaloupe	1/4 cantaloupe	=.086 mg
blackstrap molasses	1 tbsp	=.054 mg

Recommendations

• Small amounts of paprika stimulate the appetite. It is a relatively mild flavoring which goes really well with potatoes and simple casseroles whose bland textures are easiest to keep down during this time. Onions and fresh watercress also increase appetite.

• Several herbal teas having a soothing effect on digestion and appetite. Some herbal ingredients repeatedly recommended to ease nausea during pregnancy are red raspberry leaves, cinnamon, wild yam root and ginger root.

• Don't get hungry! Eating frequently in small amounts is the easiest on a roiling digestive tract and keeps digestive juices at work on food rather than the walls of your stomach.

• Oatmeal and other cooked cereals are nutritious, easy-to-digest foods. Complex carbohydrates and protein foods stay in your stomach longer, digesting more slowly than simple carbohydrates (sugars) and providing more of a buffer against active stomach acids.

• If you are likely to feel nauseous upon waking, keep crackers next to your bed and, before getting up, eat a couple slowly to soak up excess acids.

• A deficiency of vitamin B_6 produces symptoms resembling morning sickness, so check your daily B_6 intake to make sure it is at least 2.2 mg.

• Recent studies have shown that acupressure can reduce morning sickness in a majority of cases without side effects. Located on the inside forearm about $1^1/_4$ inches above the first wrist line, the pressure point is called the Neiguan Point. A product called the Sea Band—a wrist band that applies the correct amount of pressure—was reported effective in two-thirds of the women experiencing nausea, according to a recent report in the *Journal of Obstetrics and Gynecology*. The Sea Band was developed in England, and is distributed by Travel Accessories in Solon, Ohio, (216) 248-8432.

Further Information

• "Biologists Advise Doctors to Think Like Darwin" by Natalie Angier, *The New York Times*, p. C-1, December 24, 1991.

• "Easing Severe Morning Sickness: A vitamin therapy for expectant mothers" by Diana Willensky, *American Health*, Sept. 1992, p. 86.

• *Healing Yourself During Pregnancy* by Joy Gardner, Crossing Press, Freedom, CA, 1987.
• *Let's Have Healthy Children* by Adele Davis, New American Library, New York, NY, 1972.
• "Morning-Sickness Aid" by Jane Brody, *The New York Times*, p. C-18, November 18, 1992.
• *The Wise Woman Herbal for the Childbearing Year* by Susun S. Weed, Ash Tree Publishing, PO Box 64, Woodstock, NY 12498, 1986.

PROTEIN COMPLEMENTING

Although adequate protein intake is no longer reported as a problem among vegetarians, a common misconception still prevails that it is hard for vegetarians to get enough "complete" protein. This myth has been exacerbated by another one—the necessity of intricate food combining to achieve a balanced protein—introduced by Frances Moore Lappé in her book, *Diet for a Small Planet* and widely accepted. But in her 25th-anniversary edition, Lappé herself admits that she was mistaken in earlier editions of the book:

"In 1971 I stressed protein complementarity because I assumed that the only way to get enough protein (without consuming too many calories) was to create a protein as usable by the body as animal protein. In combating the myth that meat is the only way to get high-quality protein, I reinforced another myth. I gave the impression that in order to get enough protein without meat, considerable care was needed in choosing foods. Actually, it is much easier than I thought."

Her original theory regarding protein balancing suggested that grains and legumes are composed of incomplete proteins which must be combined to achieve a delicate balance of amino acids for a healthy diet. In fact, this is true of only two vegetable foods:

1. Corn, which is deficient in (but not totally lacking) the amino acid tryptophan

2. Cassava, a root vegetable which is deficient in (but not totally lacking) methionine

Fruit is the only major food group that is short on some of the amino acids (but not all). Legumes, grains and vegetables all provide adequately balanced protein. An examination of the amino acid balance of meats suggests that a high level of animal foods in the diet can create dangerous levels of the sulfur amino acids such as methionine and cystine.

Recent studies suggest that protein quality is increased by the addition of "complementary" protein foods, even if those foods are eaten as much as 16 hours before or afterwards. If you eat from all food groups every day, then you automatically increase the protein balance of all foods which are adequate to start with as well as raising the protein levels of other foods which may have a lower protein quality level by themselves. If you get sufficient calories, you are getting enough protein, provided the calories are not from junk foods. If you do not limit yourself to a single protein source, protein intake will be at least at the National Research Council's recommended dietary level (which, by the way, is higher than the Canadian recommended level, and higher than that recommended by the World Health Organization).

The strange myth of the difficulty of obtaining adequate protein from vegetable foods has its seed of truth in the diets of poor countries and perhaps in some vegetarian diets consumed during the early 1960s in the United States. In both cases, the diets were limited in carbohydrates. When insufficient carbohydrates are taken in, the body uses protein for its energy needs instead. This decreases available protein needed for healthy body maintenance and creation of new life. Fortunately, healthy carbohydrates have regained their good image, as a natural and important highlight in the diet that should not be forgotten. If you are vegetarian and get sufficient complex carbohydrates, you do not have to worry about protein intake, even when you are pregnant.

Food labeling standards of the U.S. Food and Drug Administration (USFDA) now reflect this new understanding of plant proteins. The previous FDA standards were based upon milk (casein) protein which is much richer in amino acids than necessary. Isolated soy protein is now considered ideal, and most vegetable proteins are listed as being good protein sources.

Recommendations

• Make sure you eat plenty of healthy carbohydrates (legumes, whole grains) and you will not have a protein deficiency. Another way of thinking about this is: get enough (healthy) calories in your daily diet to support adequate weight gain (at least 25 pounds) over your pregnancy. Keeping track of your own weight gain with a midwife or doctor will monitor whether your caloric intake is adequate. If it is, you are getting enough protein, provided you are not eating empty calories (junk foods).

• A diet can be protein-rich without meat or dairy products. A diet that has the 60 to 70 percent protein quality value recommended by the U.S. Food and Nutrition Board can easily be met by including foods such as black beans, pinto beans, barley, tahini, hummus, buckwheat, oats, rice, rye, wheat, chickpeas, lima beans, peas, soybeans, and any soy products such as soy milk, soy yogurt, soy flour and tofu.

Further Information

• *Amazing Grains* by Joanne Saltzman, H. J. Kramer Inc., Tiburon, CA, 1992.

• *Diet for a Small Planet* by Frances Moore Lappé, Ballantine Books, New York, NY, 1990.

• "Digestibility of Legume Proteins" by S. Suzanne Nielsen, *Food Technology*, Sept. 1991, p. 112-118.

- "Laying Down the Law on Protein" by Sally Hayhow Cullen, *Vegetarian Times,* Sept. 1992.
- *Transition to Vegetarianism* by Rudolph Ballentine, Himalayan International Institute, Honesdale, PA, 1987.
- *TVP Cookbook: Using the Quick Cooking Meat Substitutes* by Dorothy R. Bates, The Book Publishing Company, Summertown, TN, 1991.

Personal Experiences

Carmela Gustafson

Ten years a vegetarian and pregnant with my first child, I had kitchen shelves lined with Mason jars full of dried kidney, garbanzo and soy beans, lentils and split peas, kasha and barley, and brown, white and basmati rice. I had learned to cook with tofu, gluten and TVP; homemade breads and muffins rounded out the protein in my diet. By then my diet had become a way of life: the foods I ate were the ones I craved.

Although I had given up on conscious protein complementation early on (it seemed to me that variety and good sense were all I needed to insure good nutrition), I found myself thinking about and seeking out proteins more often during my pregnancy. At first, I drank a powdered protein shake for breakfast, but soon found that regular hot cereals, cottage cheese or even peanut butter served me equally well.

Debra Newby

Becoming a vegetarian during my second pregnancy was very easy for me. It was a relief not to have to gag down meat anymore in the name of getting "healthy protein." However, I still heard the voice of my doctor from my first pregnancy telling me to eat lots of protein (meat and eggs, of course) so that I would have a healthy baby. I added a lot of tofu and nut butters to my well-rounded diet of fruit, vegetables and grains. I concentrated on eating a lot of vegetable protein, probably more than I really needed to. I never told my doctor about being a vegetarian because I realized that

I probably knew more about vegetarian nutrition than he did. After nine fairly easy months and a drug-free labor, I gave birth to a beautiful, healthy boy.

Mary Halter Petersen

During my third pregnancy, I was a vegetarian. I didn't worry about protein combinations since I was aware of the latest research that shows our bodies have their own wisdom and can make complete proteins from the components of several meals. During the first few months of pregnancy and for several weeks postpartum I craved eggs, so I ate those along with my otherwise grain- and vegetable-based diet. The only dairy I ate was an occasional yogurt, which made me feel foggy, so I eventually stopped eating even that. I was healthy and strong throughout the pregnancy, and my diet supplied all the nutrients I and my baby needed. I felt better during this pregnancy than with the first two. My labor was much easier and my daughter's complexion was smoother and clearer than my first two. She is now a year old and weighs 20 pounds!

SALT

Sufficient sodium intake is essential to a healthy pregnancy. While this does not necessarily mean sufficient *salt* is essential to a healthy pregnancy, it is important to be aware of your sodium intake during this time.

The sodium content of processed foods is extremely high, but most vegetarians prefer to eat minimally processed foods: whole grains, legumes, fresh fruit and vegetables in contrast to packaged meat slices, microwaveable meals and junk foods. Most of the dire warnings about excess sodium/salt intake are directed at people in the United States who have access to and eat large quantities of processed foods. (See "Understanding Nutrients: Sodium")

In fact, macrobiotic vegetarians often avoid salt as if they were on a salt-restricted diet. U.S. macrobiotic followers, in particular, are frequently told to reduce salt as a balance for their yang tendencies. Sometimes in the U.S., this has been taken to mean that no salt is best, but traditional macrobiotic recipes often include salt.

Pregnant macrobiotics are cautioned to include sodium in their diet during pregnancy. Sea vegetables, a common part of many macrobiotic diets, are high in sodium. Additional miso and shoyu in macrobiotic dishes are traditional ways to increase dietary sodium without having to ingest table salt. (See "Macrobiotic Pregnancy")

Changes in the way things taste during pregnancy are legendary. A 1986 study by Brown and Toma, reported in the *American Journal of Nutrition,* found that pregnant women preferred and could more accurately discern the taste of stronger salt solutions than non-pregnant women. This sensitivity disappeared about six months after giving birth. If you have a craving for junk foods, it may indicate a need for more sodium; providing this essential nutrient through miso soups and salad dressings, sea salt and sea vegetables may help reduce a desire for highly processed foods.

Since excess sodium is excreted in the urine, it is also important to drink plenty of fluids (at least eight glasses a day) during pregnancy. A natural edema (water retention) occurs during pregnancy that should never be treated by reducing salt or fluids. This may run counter to a cultural dictum that salt is "bad" or a "logical" impression that water retention can be cured by reducing water intake, but please remember that with sufficient water and sodium in the diet, pregnancy establishes its own balance, one that will be healthy for the mother and the baby.

Edema, or swelling due to water retention, should of course be monitored: there is a difference between a mild, natural edema, which is barely visible, and edema which is visible and may be an early warning signal of toxemia. Also, sufficient sodium in the diet does not mean oversalting foods or eating processed foods "for the sodium content"—moderation is the rule, and extremes of avoidance or overindulgence are to be avoided.

Recommendations

• Drink at least eight glasses of water, fruit or vegetable juices every day. Most vegetables and fruits naturally contain small amounts of sodium, as do nut and soy milks.

• A recommended minimum sodium intake is set at two to three grams/day, and over 14-16 grams of sodium chloride (salt) a day is considered excessive.

• Eat sodium-rich foods such as sea vegetables (especially kelp) and foods with miso instead of table salt. While many people find sea salt will not satisfy their taste for salt, these foods do.

Further Information

• "Salt: Some Concerns" by Don Mastesz, *Macrobiotics Today*, May/June 1992, p. 27-29.

• "Salt in Cooking: How Much is Right?" by Cindy Briscoe, *Macrobiotics Today*, May/June 1992, p. 30-31.

• "Taste changes during pregnancy" by J.E. Brown and R.B. Toma, *American Journal of Nutrition*, 1986;43:414-18.

SENSORY CHANGES

Hormones are key factors in how we perceive the world through our senses. These chemical substances are produced in the adrenal glands, the pituitary gland, the thyroid glands, the testes (in men) and the ovaries (in women). Hormones act as messengers between the different systems of the body, regulating metabolism, growth, stress reactions and blood composition.

During pregnancy, the placenta becomes the most active organ in the body in terms of regulating hormones, producing extra progesterone and estrogen which, in turn, cause the bodily changes that facilitate a flourishing pregnancy.

Changes in taste, smell, hearing, vision and touch occur during pregnancy as a result of these hormonal changes, although the direct relationship has not yet been fully defined. Some women find these differences remarkable, while others barely notice them in the midst of the other physical changes of pregnancy. Sometimes the shifts create new cravings and aversions to particular foods. Aversion to the sight, smell and taste of meat is one of the most common of these, experienced in all cultures and seemingly unrelated to one's non-pregnant attitudes toward meat. (See "Cravings and Aversions")

Taste

Pregnancy brings a slight dulling of the taste buds, lowering the thresholds of taste so that it may take a stronger flavor to make an impression. Delicately seasoned foods may taste bland, spicier foods may taste just right. Often cravings arise for spicy foods: your taste buds may be calling out for sensation! There are many reports of pica, in which non-food items such as clay and starch are eaten, which surely requires a desensitization of taste.

These changes in taste most likely evolved to allow pregnant women to eat a wider variety of foods and to meet their growing appetites, which support a growing baby. For example, the slight bitterness of cruciferous vegetables, such as broccoli, Brussels sprouts, cabbage and cauliflower may be less noticeable during pregnancy. These foods are especially good for you and your baby, therefore, in this case, a perception of blander taste may be encouraging you to eat more.

A relative insensitivity to the taste of salt may also encourage the intake of more sodium which is essential to balance the increase in body fluids. This works in conjunction with another effect of progesterone during pregnancy: an increase in the rate of excretion of sodium. These two processes allow greater availability of sodium without letting it build up internally.

Smell
Women often notice a heightened sense of smell during pregnancy, along with a general increase in awareness of body sensations. Nutritionally, this change in odor perception appears to make women want to avoid most strong smells. This may provide a warning system, so that less sensitive taste buds won't let a woman eat spoiled or overly spicy foods that could be harmful to her and the growing fetus.

Vision
Sometimes women find that the sight of certain foods, particularly meat, are abhorrent during pregnancy even if they had been tolerable before. This may provide yet another warning to women to avoid potentially toxic foods even if they don't smell or taste bad. (See "Meat and Meat Hazards")

Other visual changes of pregnancy include seeing spots or lights, and double vision. These are common but should be noted because they can be a warning signal of pre-eclampsia. (See "Toxemia")

Touch and Hearing
Although a heightened awareness of one's body and a more accurate sense of hearing sometimes occur during pregnancy, these changes do not have obvious nutritional implications. They may provide the woman with more alertness during a time when progesterone is working to relax and slow the muscles of the body.

Factors likely to affect food intake
Several physiological factors will affect a pregnant woman's appetite. Placental hormones, fetal nutrient needs,

a reduction in physical activity and increase in energy needs due to increasing maternal weight are the major causes of changes in appetite.

Plasma levels of progesterone and estrogen increase throughout the mother's pregnancy. These hormones have been linked to appetite regulation in non-pregnant women via experiments which suggest that progesterone stimulates appetite while estrogen may inhibit or depress it.

During the first half of pregnancy, progesterone levels rise faster and earlier than estrogen levels, with the reverse being true during the last months of pregnancy. This is one possible explanation of why appetite and food intake increase during early pregnancy and tend to decline during the last trimester.

Energy requirements also change during pregnancy. As might be expected, the more you use up energy, the bigger your appetite. Being pregnant takes energy and so the energy requirement goes up. A greater appetite is the natural response to replenishing energy as well as generating additional energy supplies. It must be noted, however, that pregnant women tend to slow down their physical exercise as well, thus using less energy and perhaps leaving more available for the fetus.

A 1935 study by Hansen and Langer reported that the thresholds for salt, sweet, sour and bitter all increased during pregnancy, attributable to increased progesterone levels. These changes in taste receptivity may cause or abet food cravings and aversions during this time.

While the thresholds for taste increase during pregnancy, thresholds for smell decrease. Thus foods that are spicy may taste better, but foods that smell stronger do not.

Further Information
  • "Taste changes during pregnancy" by J.E. Brown and R.B. Toma, *American Journal of Nutrition*, 1986, 43:414-48.

• "Change of taste in pregnancy" by R. Hansen and W. Langer, reported in *Nutrition and Metabolism in Pregnancy* by Pedro Rosso, Oxford University Press, New York, NY, 1990.

Recommendations

• Sensory changes during pregnancy can be taken into consideration when choosing foods to prepare and eat. Working with your senses instead of trying to override them will help digestion and your overall feeling about food.

• See "Cravings and Aversions" for more specifics about changes in taste preferences.

SKIN CHANGES

Hormonal changes occur during pregnancy that can affect a woman's skin. Because of the additional progesterone, a woman is likely to find her skin somewhat more oily. This is to help the skin become flexible enough to stretch around the belly and breasts as pregnancy progresses and a woman gains weight. Rubbing vitamin E oil on these areas may be enough to prevent stretch marks.

Hormones can also affect skin color during pregnancy, depositing extra melanin in areas such as the nipples, darkening the areola. Some fair-skinned women notice a brown streak up the center of their abdomen. Most of these changes will revert after pregnancy.

During pregnancy the skin is more sensitive to the sun, also a side effect of hormonal changes. It is possible that the extra melanin is made available, on some level, to the entire body, to help counteract this sensitivity. Skin weakened through hormonal sensitivity to the sun may be more vulnerable to varicose veins, so any additional protection through extra melanin would be useful.

Skin discoloration may also be an early symptom of a folic acid or PABA deficiency (See "Understanding Nutrients: Para-Aminobenzoic Acid"), so check the level of these nutrients in your diet if unusual brown spots start appearing on your skin. Nutritional yeast, wheat germ, molasses, whole grains, fresh fruits and vegetables are rich in natural folic acid and should be added to the diet before any folic acid supplementation as a response to skin discoloration (always speak to your medical advisor/doctor before increasing levels of supplements during pregnancy). (See "Supplements")

Recommendations

• Rub vitamin E or some other gentle oil on skin that is stretching during pregnancy, particularly the abdominal area and the breasts. This will help prevent stretch marks. Applying oil on the perineum before and during labor will help prevent tearing during birth, giving more elasticity to the skin.

• Don't spend a lot of time unprotected in the sun.

• Check for a folic acid or PABA deficiency. Add foods rich in these nutrients, such as whole grains, wheat germ, and molasses to your diet, and check with your midwife/doctor if you suspect a deficiency might be causing skin discoloration.

SOCIAL PRESSURE

With the onset of pregnancy, almost every woman finds her life filled with questions but, in a meat-centered culture, pregnant vegetarians have a special set all their own. These questions come from within—What if my partner is not a vegetarian? What if my family thinks being a vegetarian is frightening? What if my doctor tells me to eat meat?—and they come from without—Don't you have to eat meat during pregnancy? Isn't it unhealthy to be a vegetarian if you are pregnant? Are you crazy?

In fact, many vegetarian women remark that pregnancy seems to be a time when even strangers who know nothing about nutrition or vegetarianism seem to feel they can offer opinions on diet—unasked.

It is hard to remember that, while such questions and opinions spring from ignorance, they are usually well-intentioned. Everyone wants a baby to be healthy when it is born and almost everyone has culturally ingrained ideas of what is essential to a healthy pregnancy. But it becomes very difficult and unpleasant to have people repeatedly say that you are not doing the best thing for your baby, no matter how self-confident you may be.

We've all heard the old adage—"Sticks and stones will break your bones, but names will never hurt you." It was supposed to help protect us from verbal bullies when we were kids. But linguist Suzette Haden Elgin was one of the first people to point out that this saying is not true. Most people have wound up feeling bad and hurt after a "mere" conversation, at least once in a while.

Elgin has developed a method, the "Gentle Art of Verbal Self-Defense," which offers tools for dealing with people who say unkind things in the guise of friendly remarks. Although not directed at vegetarians *per se,* her ideas apply to the common experience in a vegetarian pregnancy when friends, relatives and people from the medical profession make remarks that are presumably well meant, but that leave you feeling anxious about your health or your baby's.

One of the principles involved in verbal self-defense is that of a presupposition. Although not stated directly, a comment assumes certain attitudes. In the case of a pregnant vegetarian, a speaker's disapproval of your vegetarianism will be implied, but not necessarily spoken outright. For example, in the question "Do you really think it's safe to be a vegetarian while you are pregnant?", the presuppositions are that:

1. It's not really safe.
2. You can't really think it's safe.
3. If you think it's safe, you are wrong and you are not being a good mother.

You may want to respond that it *is* safe, and cite your reasons, but in doing that you must disagree with this person about a basic supposition she has made. You are in a bind: you really do think it is safe, but unless you want to argue about something that probably can't be decided on a rational level, you may be left feeling angry, hurt and annoyed, and without recourse.

Someone who believes she is disapproving for your own good may have no recognition that she is attacking you, and may in fact deny that what she is saying is an attack. Phrases such as "If you *really* care about your baby's health" or "Even *you* should know that meat is necessary to a full-term pregnancy" often include an emphasis that can signal a verbal attack.

Elgin's first recommendation in verbal self-defense is to know that you are under attack so that you don't react without knowing why. Her second principle is to switch to what she calls the "Computer Mode," proffering a factual and non-emotional response rather than trying to counterattack. This will minimize the negative impulses of the conversation.

Alternatively, confronting a person in regard to the pre-supposition may be the most effective response. Once some-one realizes that she is being unsupportive, she may wish to rephrase her concerns.

Sometimes, a doctor or parent will persist in their pres-sure to make you give up a vegetarian diet. Some vegetarian mothers have felt that deception was necessary to avoid the stress of such pressure, while others find that their doctors do not even ask about diet so the pressure is avoided alto-gether. Some pregnant vegetarians find that their good health prompts medical professionals to find out more about a vegetarian diet. Even though they may not get full approval, they have contributed to the nutritional education of a local medical professional.

Resentment and even rage over disapproval of one's diet is not uncommon. Given the hormonal changes of pregnancy, a woman may find herself responding with mild irritation and tears to even the kindest criticism. In a sense, this can almost be seen as a training ground for being a mother. Trusting your own body, respecting your own needs, and believing in the verifiable healthiness of the vegetarian diet are essential to a sense of relaxed confidence during pregnancy, but they may not be easy to maintain under pressure.

Recommendations

• Talk to parents and siblings about your vegetarian diet before you become pregnant, if possible. That way, the information won't be new to them. Offering information about the health reasons for a vegetarian pregnancy may be the best way to avoid having an emotional discussion based on misinformation.

• Talk to other vegetarians for support. Find out if any of the available doctors/midwives are vegetarians, or at least if they accept vegetarian diets as healthy. This is worth asking about before you choose a doctor. A doctor who is in favor of your dietary choices is a major source of support, and doubting relatives, friends and acquaintances will often calm down when they find you have a medical okay.

• Trust your own body. If you feel fine and have the signs of good health (proper weight gain, good appetite, healthy complexion and sufficient energy), there is no reason to give in to social pressure based on ignorance or lack of experience.

• Of course, a vegetarian partner/spouse is the strongest ally one can have. Not only will your partner be a buffer against some of the social pressure you may encounter, but you will be able to have healthy vegetarian meals prepared for you and eaten with you. If your partner/spouse is against your vegetarian diet, talk it over until you can reach an agreement of acceptance—as much as possible—before your pregnancy begins.

• Chart your daily food intake to assure and/or remind yourself that your nutrient intakes are sufficient. (See "Food Groups, Dietary Plans and RDAs") This information can also be used to assure others that you know what you are doing and are perfectly capable of having a healthy vegetarian diet that meets nutritional guidelines.

Further Information

• *The Gentle Art of Verbal Self-Defense* by Suzette Haden Elgin, Prentice Hall, New York, NY, 1980. (Elgin also has several follow-up books on the same subject: *More on the Gentle Art of Verbal Self-Defense* (1983), *Success with the Gentle Art of Verbal Self-Defense* (1987), and *The Last Word on the Gentle Art of Verbal Self-Defense* (1989).)

• *The Vegetarian Self-Defense Manual* , by Richard Bargen, Quest Books, Wheaton, IL, 1979.

• *Vegan Nutrition: A Survey of Research* by Gill Langley, The Vegan Society, London, England, 1988.

Published research supporting vegetarian diets may not be easily available in your community, but the following studies are important references to offer anyone doubting the healthiness of a vegetarian diet:

• "Health aspects of vegetarian diets" by Johanna T. Dwyer, *American Journal of Clinical Nutrition*, 1988,48:712-738. (Includes the conclusion that most vegetarian diets compare well in their adequacy, variety, balance and moderation with non-vegetarians diets and, in fact, are more in line with current dietary recommendations for nutrient intakes than meat-centered diets.)

• "Vegetarian diets—technical support paper" by the American Dietetic Association, *ADA Reports*, 1988; 88:3:352-355. (Includes a position statement that well-planned vegetarian diets effectively meet the Recommended Dietary Allowances and can be confidently embraced as a healthy dietary alternative.)

In addition, the good health of vegetarian children has been repeatedly reported by researchers, which may be of additional reassurance. A complete look at research on the health status of vegetarian children is also available in my book *Vegetarian Children* (McBooks Press, 1987, Chapter 3).

• "Mental Age and IQ of Predominantly Vegetarian Children" by Johanna T. Dwyer *et al.*, *Journal of the American Dietetic Association*, 1980, 76:142-147. (A report that vegetarian children tended to be smarter than non-vegetarian children. However, a generally higher level of nutritional knowledge among vegetarian parents may have accounted for the superior diets of the vegetarian children.)
• "Growth in 'New' Vegetarian Preschool Children using the Jenss-Bayley Curve Fitting Technique" by Johanna T. Dwyer, *et al.*, *American Journal of Clinical Nutrition*, 1983, 37:815-827. (A report that vegetarian children tended to be as tall or taller than non-vegetarian children, indicating that fears about "smaller" vegetarian children are unfounded.)

Personal Experiences
Caroline Ziogas
A few months after I turned 17, I became pregnant. My husband also decided to become a vegetarian during this time and was very supportive. When my doctor found out I was a vegetarian, she had me visit a dietitian who turned out to be most helpful and concerned. The dietitian gave me a reprint

of an article called "Vegetarian Nutrition" and recommended the books, *Laurel's Kitchen* and *Diet for a Small Planet.*

When I asked the dietitian what was most important to pay attention to, she said "Calcium and protein," and recommended I try to consume 100 grams of protein a day. She suggested I log what I ate day to day, so that she and my doctor could check it. I learned to be careful about proteins. I never felt any criticism from either my dietitian or my doctor as they gave me the information I needed.

Stephanie Ingram

At the local health department where I have been going for prenatal care, I exhaust the staff with my unending questions. I am the first vegan they have ever met there. The staff all like me and are intrigued by my choices, but also think I'm a little crazy to take a chance with a diet they know nothing about.

I have explained to them that I use soy and rice milks in my diet and that, like those with lactose intolerance, I don't eat cheese. The nutritionist had never heard of soy or rice milk, soy cheese or tofu ice cream. She was very alarmed when I told her I was drinking red raspberry leaf tea, and asked me to stick to apple juice or some frozen concentrate.

I soon understood that the extent of her nutrition education was very limited. My enjoyment and health from eating an animal-free diet confused her. Once, as I was leaving her small office, she requested that I bring a sample of my soy milk to my next visit. Happily, I agreed. The doctors and nurses have started to applaud my health status, attitude and interest in the whole baby experience.

Julie A. Prychitko

During my 23rd week of pregnancy, my husband and I attended the baptism of a friend's baby. I was stuffed with salads, vegetables, lasagna, eggplant parmesan and cake by the end of the baptismal party, when Aunt Mary introduced herself to me. She said something like, "Hi, I'm Aunt Mary. It was nice meeting you (we had just met that moment). Give me a hug. So, you're a vegetarian . . . what do you eat?" As I pointed out the many delicious Italian entrees I had just eaten, I noticed that all eyes were on me. Several of the elderly women had quite a discussion about my apparently radical eating choices during pregnancy. But they all wished me good luck as they left the party.

Deborah Aldrich

It wasn't until my first visit to the gynecologist that it ever occurred to me that it might be unusual for a pregnant woman to be a vegetarian. Karen, a midwife working for the gynecologist, began what turned out to be a series of lectures on the dangers of vegetarianism during pregnancy. She was convinced that if I didn't follow the Federal Food and Drug Administration's recommendations for pregnant women, I was endangering the health of myself and my baby. That meant eating three servings of meat and four servings of milk every day. Karen wasn't the only one to strongly object to a vegetarian diet. My "boss" (the mother of the two children I took care of) said, "You can't be a vegetarian if you're pregnant!"

Devorah L. Knaff

One difficult aspect of my vegetarian pregnancy which I dealt with daily was how friends, acquaintances and family members reacted to my diet. People I had known for years and who had ignored my eating habits suddenly displayed the urge to criticize me. "Are you *sure* you're getting enough protein/vitamins/calcium, etc.?" people frequently asked. One person actually said, in dark tones, "Something might happen to the fetus and you would always have to wonder if your diet didn't have something to do with it."

I sometimes felt something very close to rage at these comments: I knew my diet was much healthier than theirs or those of most pregnant women. I resented the fact that, as soon as a woman becomes pregnant, people feel free to treat her body and habits as public property.

SUPPLEMENTS

Taking supplements is a controversial issue. Many people take *some* vitamin and mineral supplements on a regular basis and don't think twice about it— 40 to 60 percent of adults in the U.S., according to a November 1991 report from the American Dietetic Association. Some people I know (who are generally healthy) take more than 10 pill supplements at least once a day. Many people still believe that "more is better"—that megadoses of nutrients will make you even healthier. But some vitamins and minerals are lethal in high dosages. Pregnant women should be aware that, passed along to the fetus, such high dosages can cause damage in the developmental process.

Other people avoid supplements completely, believing that eating whole foods is the only way to get proper nutrients. However, at times, limited supplementation is helpful. If nutritional demands cannot be met because of diet or metabolism, the health of the baby and the mother can be increased by specific supplementation, particularly in the cases of folic acid and iron. During pregnancy, supplements are routinely recommended.

The Institute of Medicine in Washington DC studied supplement use during pregnancy because of the dangers of both over- and under-dosing. They maintained that food is "the normal vehicle for delivering nutrients, and nutrient supplementation is an intervention," with possibly harmful effects (1990).

The American College of Obstetricians and Gynecologists recommended supplementation during pregnancy in the situation where increased needs for protein, iron, folic acid and other nutrients cannot or are not being met by dietary intake (1985).

The American Dietetic Association confirmed that use of supplements is indicated for some pregnant women, although the precise recommendations should be made by physicians and registered dietitians on an individual basis (1987).

The federal Task Force on Adolescent Pregnancy specifically recommended iron and folic acid supplementation for all pregnant teenagers (1985). Certainly, these recommendations are to be taken the way the RDAs for the general population are intended: as overall guidelines, not minimal nor necessarily optimal, and always within the context of the individual pregnant woman. In addition, these recommendations are based on the 1980 RDAs, which were updated in 1989.

Most people do not reach the RDA for all nutrients. This is because the RDA is a figure designed to meet the needs of the average person. Your own RDA may not exactly match the norm. The USRDAs (used for labeling in America) are higher than the RDAs, to surpass average needs. Prescriptions for prenatal vitamin and mineral supplements are often based on the USRDA (as determined by the Food and Drug Administration).

It is very difficult to get too much of a particular vitamin or mineral if you are eating food and not taking supplements. Nutrients tend to be balanced within foods and interact in ways that are still being discovered. An imbalance caused by too great a dose of an individual nutrient can interfere with the usage of other nutrients. A supplement only contains a concoction of known nutrients, and in larger-than-life dosages. Although our bodies are good at excreting excess nutrients as waste, this is not always a foolproof system.

The range of vitamins and minerals that are available in supplement form is smaller than the range of nutrients found in whole foods. Supplements do not give you the health benefits of eating real foods: fiber, micro-nutrients and even fats are missing from supplements. Other health benefits of fresh foods may yet be discovered.

In rare situations, individual foods can be very dense in a particular nutrient which, consumed alone and in excess, could be harmful. For example, if you ate only carrots, you might develop a yellow skin discoloration associated with an overdose of Vitamin A. But if you ate other things besides carrots you would be less likely to have this reaction.

Researchers and doctors are concerned about the dangers of self-supplementation. Getting vitamin and mineral supplements, as well as more complex supplements, is easier than getting information on the safe way to use them. Health food stores always have a wide selection of supplements for every nutrient and a hundred different ailments. Anyone can go in, reacting to whatever information is available, the advertising on the supplements themselves, or articles and books they have read, and choose supplements to any desired level.

But both high and low dosages of the same nutrient can be harmful to your health. For example, a high level of folacin intake (higher than the RDA) is not beneficial because it inhibits zinc and iron absorption in the gastrointestinal tract. Since there is already a possibility of zinc deficiency in pregnancy, it is important not to overdo it on folacin.

On the other hand, too low a level of folacin during pregnancy has been linked with an increase in neural tube birth defects, such as spina bifida. So a middle ground must be reached through diet with supplementation—if dietary folacin is insufficient. (See "Understanding Nutrients: Folic Acid")

Sometimes, doctors recommend starting a folic acid supplement three months before conception, so that any deficiency can be made up ahead of time, to avoid the need for supplementation later. This principle may be applied to other supplements as well. If you use birth control pills, drink alcohol or eat an unhealthy diet, do something about it at least three to six months before you conceive so that your body will start pregnancy with good reserves of all nutrients.

Nutrient levels can be measured in a blood sample. During pregnancy the mother's body shows an enormous increase in blood volume, to provide sustenance to the baby. Even if nutrient levels do not drop, their ratio to total blood volume is likely to be reduced naturally by this expansion. Test results indicate deficiencies as a lower density or as an absolute decrease.

Prenatal nutrient tests are usually done for iron levels and, more recently, for folic acid levels as well. If you eat few or no animal products, request that your B_{12} level also be checked. (See "Understanding Nutrients: Vitamin B_{12}") Although it is unlikely to be low, B_{12} is vital to healthy fetal development and it is important to know whether your body is functioning properly on its current B_{12} intake.

Herbs and herbal supplements contain a lot of different nutrients, many of which have not been researched at all, and no Recommended Dietary Allowances for them have been made. Herb supplements should be taken with care, and used as medicines. The health branch of the U.S. federal government is beginning to understand how powerful these health food store herbal supplements are. They are currently attempting to put supplements under strict regulation to prevent abuses. I can remember when people laughed at the idea that such supplements could do anything, but now, apparently, the federal government takes them seriously enough to try to include them under prohibitive bureaucracy so that no one gets hurt (or helped) by them without official permission.

It is true that some dietary supplements can be unhealthy. Their nutrient dosages are too high because they have been marketed without research into their value and use. Or the nutrient may be packaged in an unhealthy base: calcium supplements have been known to be contaminated with high levels of lead. Because of this, it is wise to read the label carefully when choosing supplements.

Recommendations

• Read the label of a dietary or nutritional supplement to see what *all* the ingredients are. Check up on ingredient names that you don't recognize.

• Natural excesses of nutrients found in herbs (as opposed to herbal supplements where one element is isolated) are better for you than those in pill form. This is because herbs are whole foods and have additional balancing factors such as fiber, which protect the nutrient. Fresh herbs on your salad and rice dishes can usually provide all the additional nutrients that your body could need. Leeks, chives, watercress and other cresses, dandelions, chervil and spinach are some greens that are unusually nutrient-rich.

• See "Nutrients" section for limits on supplementation of individual nutrients.

Further Information

• "A Shopper's Guide to the Sensible Use of Vitamin and Mineral Supplements" by Bill Thomson, *Natural Health*, March/April 1992, 82-99.

• "Dietary Supplements: Let the Buyer Beware", by Marian Burros, *The New York Times*, October 16, 1991, p. C3.

• "Eating Well: Vitamins are fine, with the *right* foods" by Marian Burros, *The New York Times*, June 24, 1992, p. C3.

• "Forget the Prenatal Vitamins, and Eat for Two!" by Ellen Kleiner, *Mothering*, Fall 1991, 97.

• *Nutrition During Pregnancy, Part II: Nutrient Supplements* by the Institute of Medicine, National Academy Press, Washington, DC, 1990.

• "Relationship of vitamin/mineral supplements to certain psychological factors" by Marsha Read *et al.*, *Journal of the American Dietetic Association*, 1991:11:1429-1430.

Personal Experiences
Sharon K. Yntema

When I was pregnant in 1977, I didn't think twice about taking the supplements my general practitioner recommended. I figured it was better to cover the odds by having a little too much rather than too little and I never questioned it further, even to myself.

My doctor recommended four supplements: *Thera M* (a multi-vitamin/mineral supplement with 12 mg iron), *Orgd5 Iron* (75 mg with B and C vitamins), folic acid (800 mcg) and vitamin E (200 IU). I was worried about iron supplementation because although I was sure extra iron was necessary, I was given a supplement with double the RDA for iron, and I knew that extra iron often caused constipation. This was of particular concern to me in later pregnancy when constipation became more of a problem for me.

TOXEMIA

Toxemia is a term that can be used for any hypertension problem during pregnancy. It is *not* a blood disease where toxins circulate in the body, despite the way it sounds (toxi = toxin, emia = heme = blood). It is usually diagnosed in the third trimester.

If high blood pressure exists before pregnancy, it is called *chronic hypertensive vascular disease.* If blood pressure rises after conception, it is called pre-eclampsia or *pregnancy-induced hypertension.* Most mothers with chronic high blood pressure are women over 30 who have already had a child. The two kinds of hypertension (chronic and with onset after conception) require slightly different treatments.

Most pregnant women experience a slightly elevated blood pressure, which is considered normal. When blood pressure rises abruptly, or climbs above 140/90, or reaches an increase of 15 over a baseline, the condition is called *mild pre-eclampsia*. Abnormal readings must be verified on at least two occasions, about six hours apart. Mild pre-eclampsia is considered of particular concern if the rise in blood pressure occurs at the same time as edema, unusual weight gain and/or a raised level of protein in the blood where none had been present before.

If blood pressure continues to rise (over 160/110), or edema/weight gain becomes severe, the diagnosis is changed to *severe pre-eclampsia*. Medical care is essential at this point because there is danger of convulsions.

Surprisingly little is known about the causes of high blood pressure during pregnancy, but the link to nutrition is strong, just as it is in a non-pregnant person. Toxemia has been linked to a folic acid deficiency, and possibly to a sodium/potassium imbalance that can be controlled nutritionally. According to World Health Organization researchers, a 2,000 mg/day calcium supplement has been shown to help maintain normal blood pressure, but not all pregnant women were able to control their blood pressure in this way. Several studies reported in the early 1990s supported the use of calcium supplementation to control high blood pressure and possibly prevent pre-eclampsia.

Pre-eclampsia has been observed in pregnant women whose protein intake is considered abnormally low. Additionally, some pregnant women with pre-eclampsia have reduced the symptoms when their protein intake was clinically increased. This research seems to show that there is a connection between maternal protein intake and toxemia.

Because both edema (swelling of hands, ankles and feet) and unusually high sodium retention are present with toxemia, many doctors once jumped to the conclusion that reducing salt and/or fluid intake would help correct this problem. However, since higher-than-average sodium retention is not only normal but essential to a healthy pregnancy, the conclusion was wrong. In fact, reducing salt or liquids in the diet is now considered dangerous, because it will only further upset the sodium balance of the body. (See "Salt")

Edema and sudden, excessive weight gain are the result of an abnormal accumulation of water in the tissues; gains of more than three pounds a week are considered quite high. Taking diuretics, reducing salt or eating less food to lose weight are not "solutions"—they will only increase the problems of high blood pressure and edema.

Malnutrition has been linked to hypertension. Women who gain 25 to 30 pounds during their pregnancy have been found to be less likely to develop toxemia. Both too little and too much protein may aggravate hypertension, which suggests that a vegetarian diet, with its moderate approach to protein intake, may be the answer.

In fact, numerous studies have shown that a strict vegetarian diet will help control hypertension. In one study, even vegetarians who drank milk and ate eggs had lower blood pressures than meat-eaters. Some of the factors which possibly account for this connection are high-fiber diets and a high ratio of polyunsaturated to saturated fats in the diet.

Recommendations

• Avoid stimulants such as caffeine which raise blood pressure as they keep you awake.

• Get plenty of exercise. This will provide a natural massage of all body systems and help to decrease water retention as well as help stabilize your blood pressure.

• Eat calcium-rich foods such as leafy green vegetables (always eat spinach with rice which increases the bio-availability of the calcium) and tofu made with calcium silicate. (See "Nutrients: Calcium")

• Sufficient doses of vitamins C and E in the diet may be essential in the prevention of pre-eclampsia. Although supplemental doses of these antioxidants may be useful, this is still only considered a possible solution, and neither vitamin should be taken in excess without medical supervision.

• Make sure to eat plenty of vitamin C-rich fresh fruits and vegetables (at least 5 servings a day) and don't cut out cold-pressed vegetable oils. Wheat germ, nuts and seeds are also naturally rich sources of vitamin E. If you eat well, supplementation will be unnecessary.

• Raw garlic, parsley, onions, cucumber ($\frac{1}{2}$ cup juice or one cucumber daily), and celery are all folk remedies for hypertension whose value has more recently been confirmed by scientific research. Raw beet juice will improve your sodium/potassium balance as well as provide additional natural calcium. Bananas, dandelion greens and chicory are also recommended.

• Make sure you are getting at least 800 mcg of folic acid per day.

• Do not take water pills or diuretics and do not restrict your salt intake.

Further Information

• "Pregnancy-induced hypertension and low birth weight: the role of calcium" by John T. Repke and Jose Villar, *American Journal of Clinical Nutrition*, 1991, 54:2375-2415. (Suggests that lowering blood pressure through calcium supplementation may reduce the incidence of pre-eclampsia, premature birth and low birth rate.)

• "The effects of calcium supplementation on normotensive and hypertensive pregnancy" by K. B. Knight and R.E. Keith, *American Journal of Clinical Nutrition*, 1992, 55:891-95. (Recommends calcium supplements for treating high blood pressure during pregnancy.)

• "The relationship between calcium intake and pregnancy-induced hypertension: up-to-date evidence" by J.M. Belizan *et al., American Journal of Obstetrics and Gynecology*, 1988, 158:898-902.

• "Trace minerals in pregnancy" by P. Yasodhara, *et al., Nutrition Research*, 1991, 11:15-21. (Reports that lowered calcium levels are found in pregnancy-induced hypertension but not in pre-eclampsia. Lowered zinc levels are found in both situations.)

Personal Experiences
Sharon K. Yntema

During pregnancy, my blood pressure reading went up from 105/65 to 120/80. My midwife, monitoring this change, suggested I eat more protein and less salt, in hopes that it would counter an onset of pre-eclampsia. I had no sign of edema and my urine showed no sign of protein, despite the increase in my protein intake. Without two or three of the signs of toxemia, high blood pressure by itself is not pre-eclampsia, so increasing protein intake seemed to be an appropriate response. (No one really knew about the role of calcium in controlling high blood pressure at the time.)

When I went into labor, my blood pressure shot up into the dangerous zone (146/96). Although I had been planning a home birth for a year-and-a-half, the midwife said that I must go to the hospital because toxemia could develop quickly and my high blood pressure could cause labor complications.

Fortunately, this situation never became life-threatening, to either myself or my son. I ended up having a caesarean because, although I was in labor and the baby was overdue, I was not dilating; his head had not dropped down onto the cervix to encourage dilation and my bone structure was too small. I suspected my body sensed the impending possibility of life-threatening circumstances in giving birth (without a caesarean, probably neither of us could have survived), and went into a state of high stress, raising my blood pressure.

I have since determined that I have had high blood pressure readings for a good part of my life, although the readings were borderline high and always attributed to stress over being in the doctor's office. I also have several immediate family members who have had problems with high blood pressure. I now suspect that my body showed stable readings during most of my pregnancy due to my general level of health and well-being, but that my blood pressure did go up in response to the impending threat of a birth that would not have succeeded without medical intervention.

TOXINS (ENVIRONMENTAL)

Anything that can affect the mother's health can also affect the fetus. Good nutrition helps healthy development and toxins can increase the possibility of damage. Before pregnancy is the best time for you to learn about the toxins in your personal environment, and to figure out how you can clean it up. Keep in mind always that healthy babies are born all the time, in the most adverse of circumstances. But prevention never hurts, and usually increases the good odds.

There are three ways in which environmental and chemical damage occurs:

1. *Mutagenically:* the structure of the genetic material in one of the parents is permanently changed.

2. *Teratogenically:* the structure of the genetic material is damaged in the fetus but not necessarily in the mother. The fetus may then have birth defects, as cells develop abnormally.

3. *Carcinogenically/Oncogenically:* Normal cells in the parent or child begin to mutate.

One of the problems with toxins in the environment is that they are usually outside of our control. For example, toxins from industrial waste are found in the air and in our water supplies. Some of these kinds of toxins will accumulate in your body as you get older. However, recent research has shown that green vegetables, particularly broccoli, may provide a natural anti-toxin cleansing effect in the body when eaten regularly. While this will not counteract serious environmental pollution, it will help keep the body as healthy as it can be under the circumstances.

If you don't already know about the toxins which lurk almost everywhere these days, you may find the new knowledge particularly scary. Information out of perspective can sound disturbing to anyone. During pregnancy, I saw the cover of a book I'd studied in graduate school, *Is My Baby All Right?*, by Virginia Apgar and Joan Beck. It was a fascinating book in school, but my pregnant imagination took off worrying about all the possibilities of fetal damage that I could remember (which were a surprising number)!

I had to reassure myself that my chances for a healthy baby were good, especially since I was a vegetarian. Being a vegetarian meant that I had far fewer toxins from meats and non-organically grown fruits and vegetables in my body. (See "Meat and Meat Hazards") By avoiding these toxins even before conception, I had already increased the odds of having a healthy baby—and so can you.

It is important to know the general limits of what you can change and what is beyond your control. You cannot control the ozone layer by the time you get pregnant, even if you put full effort into it. A more successful response to the ozone danger has to be an international project, although each fluorocarbon-based spray product you refuse to use or buy is an important individual contribution.

You can control the kinds of home cleaners you use, avoiding those with particularly toxic fumes, and you should avoid painting, particularly without a face mask, during pregnancy. If you are interested in obtaining the safest home supplies, you can either find them locally or you can order them. I am sure there are many other qualified mail order programs, but the following companies responded to my request for information on home care products:

SUNRISE LANE
780 Greenwich Street
New York, NY 10014
(212) 242-7014
"A catalog of cruelty-free and biodegradable products for you and your home"

HUMANE ALTERNATIVE PRODUCTS
8 Hutchins Street
Concord, NH 03301
(603) 224-1361
"Fully guaranteed products without animal testing and containing no animal ingredients"

N.E.E.D.S. (National Ecological and Environmental Delivery System)
527 Charles Avenue 12-A
Syracuse, NY 13209
(800) 634-1380
"Helping to improve the quality of life for the ecologically sensitive person"

The following is a list of environmental toxins that you are likely to encounter and have the power to avoid. Take at least whatever common sense precautions you can. For example, if you need X-rays for dental work, have them done before pregnancy. If you use birth control pills or an IUD, stop their use at least three months before you get pregnant. Birth control pills affect the hormonal system, working against conception. It is best to give your body a chance to recover from this chemically induced control before the hormones of pregnancy begin their work.

Smoke
Alcohol
Radiation
Chemical stimulants and depressants
Aspirin

Antihistamines
Laxatives
Antacids
Diuretics
Hexachlorophene (as in PhisoHex)
Anti-nausea drugs
Most prescription and over-the-counter drugs
Recreational drugs
Heavy metals
Pesticides, herbicides, insecticides (especially those containing Carbaryl)

No one quite knows if computer use during pregnancy can be linked to any pregnancy or birth problems. Problems have turned up in some—but not all—offices where computers are used frequently. Radiation emissions are strongest at the sides and back of a computer rather than in the direction of the user, so if you work at a single computer in an office or home, the risk is automatically reduced. Some of the most common problems encountered by regular computer users have to do with body discomfort from long hours of work at a terminal. Be sure to sit up straight, in a chair that will provide lower back support and get up to stretch frequently.

Microwave ovens are another electronic device a pregnant woman might question. Microwaving can cook vegetables with a minimum of vitamin loss; many other foods can be cooked without the use of fats and oils by this method. Research suggests that microwaves have come a long way in safety protection since their appearance in the early 1980s.

However, any exposure to microwave radiation is potentially harmful to a fetus and until research shows a clearer lack of danger, it is probably best to keep microwave use to a minimum while you are pregnant. Additionally, be careful about the kinds of containers used since plastic containers and wrappers can leak chemicals into the food through the microwaving process. Transfer all foods to glass containers to provide the necessary safety.

For information on counteracting environmental toxins, see "Detoxification."

Further Information

• "Microwaving on the Make" by Mariclare Barrett Obis, *Vegetarian Times*, Sept. 1992, 91-93.

• *At Highest Risk* by Christopher Norwood, Penguin, New York, NY 1980.

• *Quick Harvest: A Vegetarian's Guide to Microwave Cooking* by Pat Baird, Prentice Hall, New York, NY, 1991.

• "Zapping Your Concerns" by Karin Horgan, *Vegetarian Times*, Sept. 1992, p. 92.

TOXINS (FOOD-RELATED)

Sometimes it seems as if everything has some danger and there may be some truth in that. However, the solution is to make the best of the situation with information and common sense as twin guides. Finding out the risks can be shocking and frightening, but a basic understanding is the wisest approach.

Some foods carry natural toxins, for example, the green portions of unripe potatoes, the leaves and flowers of the rhubarb plant or poisonous mushrooms. Plants, particularly root vegetables, are likely to absorb pesticides, industrial waste chemicals and toxic metals from the soil. The toxins are then transmitted when the root vegetables are eaten. This is one of the major arguments for organically grown foods: healthier soil means healthier vegetables and other plant foods.

Pesticides are sprayed on plants to protect the crop from insects and fungi. *Food preservatives* and *irradiation* are used to make sure foods store and travel well, looking their best when they finally reach their supermarket destinations. *Additives* are used to make foods more appealing to the eye through color and texture changes. Alar is one additive which became well-known when actress Meryl Streep publicly protested the use of this chemical which keeps apple texture firmer and apple color redder than it would be naturally. In fact, artificial food colorings, MSG and other flavorings may be added to foods by consumers themselves.

Sprouts are an example of a nutritious food that can carry toxins. A plant seed carries a higher percentage of contaminants from the environment than does a fully grown plant. According to an article by Andrew Weil, legumes carry some of the highest concentrations of natural and environmental toxins. He recommends avoiding legume sprouts for this reason. Legume sprouts can be used safely in soups and baked vegetable breads, because the heat neutralizes the natural toxic effects.

Weil also reports that alfalfa sprouts have a naturally occurring toxin, saponin, that increases during the sprouting process, resulting in possible damage to red blood cells. Alfalfa sprouts contain canavanine which can cause harm to the immune system. Weil recommends buckwheat, sunflower and radish sprouts as examples of non-legume sprouts that can provide the nutrients without the toxins. Sprouted breads are also good sources.

Herbs which may be medically useful to adults may be harmful to a developing baby. Herbs may be gentler than prescription medicines for easing a variety of health problems, but they are still strong and should be used selectively. For example, some herbs are likely to be toxic to the growing fetus and so should be avoided altogether by pregnant mothers. Among the herbs to avoid are:

angelica (can promote menstruation/miscarriage)
black cohosh or blue cohosh (can promote uterine contractions, increasing incidence of miscarriages)

coltsfoot (contains alkaloids that may damage the liver of
the fetus)
comfrey (contains alkaloids that may damage both maternal and fetal livers)
dong quai (can promote menstruation/miscarriage)
echinacea (a powerful medicine that may be too concentrated
for a fetus)
feverfew (can promote menstruation/miscarriage)
ginger root (can promote menstruation/miscarriage)
ginseng (can affect hormonal system during crucial stages
of fetal development)
goldenseal (can promote uterine contractions)
licorice (can affect hormonal system during crucial stages of
fetal development)
mugwort (a powerful medicine that may be too concentrated
for a fetus)
pennyroyal (can promote uterine contractions, increasing
incidence of miscarriages)
tansy (can promote menstruation/miscarriage)
valerian (a powerful medicine that may be too concentrated
for a fetus)
yarrow (a powerful medicine that may be too concentrated
for a fetus)

Vitamin and mineral supplements may be made from
unhealthy sources. (See "Supplements") For example, calcium supplements are frequently made from bone meal or
dolomite, which may contain lead, mercury, arsenic or other
metal toxins.

Recommendations
• Choose locally grown foods in season. Without trans-
portation or long-term storage, the need for preservatives
and food irradiation is greatly reduced. Economics has as
much an influence on farmers as morals in this: If there is

no need to spend the money for extra preservatives, the money won't be spent.

• Shop at local natural foods stores. If you are unsure how strict their limits are on purchasing organic foods, ask. Some stores label foods according to their level of purity. For example, a local store where I live sells both sulfurized and sulfur-free apricots, but the labeling is explicit, as it is for fresh produce.

• During the spring, summer, and often into the fall, most areas outside large cities have roadside fresh fruit and vegetable stands or farmers markets. Some of these places will use pesticides and preservatives, but others take pride in producing organically grown foods. Ask friends for recommendations of good places to shop, and ask the vendors at markets if they use pesticides, and to what extent.

• Wash foods gently but thoroughly, using a soft scrub brush on fruits and vegetables with skins. Peel the skin off fruits and vegetables that are unlikely to be organically grown. Take the outer leaves off lettuce, spinach and other leafy vegetables as they are most likely to have retained pesticide residue.

• Buy a minimum of processed foods. This automatically reduces the chemicals found in your meals. Organically grown legumes, rice and other dried goods can be obtained through mail order stores. An up-to-date listing of available sources for these foods can be found in the back of any health-related magazine: *Vegetarian Times, Natural Health, New Age Journal* and the like.

• Use natural dyes from plant sources such as beets, grape skins, saffron and cranberries instead of artificial food colorings. Flavor things with organically produced spices; the commercially produced ones are as likely to contain pesticide residue as the plants from which they come.

• Grow your own herbs and spices, vegetables and fruits, to whatever extent possible. If you live in a city, you may have friends or fellow workers who live in the country and have excess produce they will give or sell to you inexpensively. Some smaller cities have community gardens where space and technical assistance are provided so that residents can grow food even without land of their own.

• Remember that, although it may be impossible to avoid all pesticides, eating fresh vegetables and fruits that you have washed is preferable to avoiding these foods as a way to reduce your exposure. Some foods, such as broccoli, collard greens, kale and other green leafy vegetables provide nutritional protection against many environmentally produced toxins.

• Finally, to no one's great surprise who is reading this book, reducing intake of animal foods, including milk, is one of the most effective ways to reduce intake of toxins through foods. (See "Meat and Meat Hazards, Milk, Dairy and Eggs")

Further Information

• "Are Sprouts Health Foods? Naturally occurring toxins create doubts" by Andrew Weil, *Natural Health*, Nov/Dec, 1992.

• *Diet for a Poisoned World* by David Steinman, Ballantine Books, New York, NY, 1990.

• *Midwifery and Herbs* by Willa Shaffer, Woodland Books, PO Box 1142, Provo, Utah 84603, 1986.

• *Safe Food: Eating Wisely In a Risky World* by Michael F. Jacobson, Living Planet Press, Venice, CA. 1991.

• *The A to Z Guide to Toxic Foods and How to Avoid Them* by Lynn T. Sonberg, Pocket Books, New York, NY, 1992.

• *The Wise Woman Herbal for the Childbearing Year* by Susun S. Weed, Ash Tree Publishing, PO Box 64, Woodstock, NY 12498, 1986.

• "Warning: Avoid These Herbs During Pregnancy" by Paul Bergner, *Natural Health* , Jul/Aug, 1992, 58-62.

VARICOSE VEINS

Veins that have become swollen or dilated are called varicose veins. They usually occur in the legs because of the gravitational pressure on blood going through the legs as they support the body. Veins nearest the surface tend to have the weakest walls and no support from muscles in retaining their normal size, as deeper veins might have.

With the additional weight of pregnancy, pressure on the leg veins increases and varicose veins become more likely. However, some evidence shows that a vegetarian diet is associated with a lower incidence of varicose veins, possibly because of the role of fiber in body health.

Fiber in the diet keeps stool soft. Soft stool not only reduces the chance of hemorrhoids from straining against constipation, but also allows maximum room for an even blood flow throughout the body. Uneven and blocked blood flow combined with the pressure of pregnant abdominal weight will increase the chances of getting varicose veins (and hemorrhoids).

Recommendations

• Be sure to get regular exercise without straining your body too much.

• Give your legs a rest every day. This means putting your feet above the level of your chest which eases the pressures of additional body weight and gravity at the same time. Expansion of the pelvic bone area tends to cause a cramping of blood flow to the legs, so this simple prevention is very important.

• Don't strain on the toilet. This will protect against hemorrhoids as well.

• Eat raw fruits and vegetables and whole grain foods. This might be a tough recommendation to many meat-eaters, but vegetarians eat a much higher percentage of fiber in their diet. A report in *The Journal of the Royal Society of Health* (vol. 105, 1985) found that the vegetarians studied (who had been vegetarians for most, if not all of their lives) had fewer problems with varicose veins than non-vegetarians.

• Avoid a lot of sunlight: exposure may weaken the skin's strength in supporting the veins. Without support, the veins can become engorged (varicose).

• Hosiery has been developed to provide extra support for the veins of your legs. Although it may seem mostly like a marketing gimmick, support stockings can be helpful during pregnancy.

VEGAN PREGNANCY

Vegans by definition do not eat any animal foods, including milk, dairy and eggs. While other vegetarians may eat animal products which do not involve damage or death to the originating animal, vegans will not. The definition in Debra Wasserman's important book, *Simply Vegan*, explains that vegans do not eat milk, dairy, eggs or honey, and also do not use animal products such as leather goods, or body care items which require animal ingredients.

Lacto-ovo vegetarian diets are officially accepted as healthy, perhaps even preferable to meat-centered diets, by major medical institutions such as the American Dietetic Association and the National Academy of Sciences. But vegan diets are still portrayed in the public culture as questionable. That question is primarily one of ignorance, but it is pervasive in this meat-eating culture. (See "Social Pressure")

Because vegans do not eat cheese and eggs or drink milk, they may have a calcium deficiency if their diet does not include other calcium-rich foods such as sesame and soy milks and spreads, dark green vegetables and blackstrap molasses. (See "Understanding Nutrients: Calcium") Lactose-intolerant people have the same need to include other calcium-rich foods in their diets since they cannot digest milk properly. If your doctor is concerned about your calcium intake because you are a vegan, ask about lactose-intolerant diets; this may be a comfortable analogy for someone who is not knowledgeable about vegan diets.

Vitamin D is sometimes considered a risk factor for vegans, since most dietary vitamin D in the U.S. is consumed through fortified milk. (See "Important Nutients: Vitamin D") Pregnant vegans who live in very cloudy areas and are not exposed to sunlight for at least 15 minutes a day (face and arms) should consider a vitamin D supplement (note: vitamin D supplements can be derived from animal or vegetable matter, so check the labels on the bottles).

Vitamin B_{12} is only made from animal sources, albeit on the level of bacteria, and therefore could be said to be available from animal foods only. A simple blood test, the radioassay, can be done to determine vitamin B_{12} levels, but it may not be entirely reliable. Still, vitamin B_{12}-fortified foods (such as brewer's yeast) or a B_{12} supplement are recommended for vegans during pregnancy, even by vegan nutritionists.

Some research suggests that B_{12} can be stored in the body for years (e.g., from a previous meat-eating diet), that bacteria in the human body can manufacture this vitamin in the intestines, and that B_{12} can be found in some edible sea plant sources. While some or all of these factors may be true, none can be used consistently to assure adequate B_{12} in the diet during the crucial development of pregnancy.

Animal foods, particularly milk, cheeses and yogurt, add carbohydrates to the diet. Since an increase in carbohydrate intake is essential during pregnancy, the medical profession frequently worries that vegans will have inadequate amounts of this essential nutrient. In general, studies of vegan children show that the babies are smaller and shorter at birth than children of lacto-ovo vegetarians, a fact which probably reflects the vegans' commonly lower carbohydrate intake.

It may seem difficult for a vegan to consume enough carbohydrates in plant foods to meet the recommended daily requirement during pregnancy (determined by rate and amount of increase in maternal weight from conception to term). But natural increases in appetite provide the desire to eat more, and vegans should feel free to eat frequently and to capacity. Don't feel bothered if your medical advisor is concerned about less than average weight gain. Babies that are larger at birth have fewer developmental and health problems than undersized babies.

Vegan diets are lower in fats and have been associated with a lowered incidence of blood pressure, cholesterol, heart problems and osteoporosis. Pre-eclampsia was found to be much less frequent in pregnant vegan women and recent studies are showing that vegan children are healthy and thriving.

A vegan diet during pregnancy requires extra attention to the nutrients mentioned above, particularly in our meat-oriented society, which does not provide proper nutrition education and support to vegan families. This extra time and attention may not be possible and some pregnant vegans add occasional eggs, milk, and yogurt to their diets for assurance. It is important for these women not to blame themselves for temporarily changing from their ideal diet, because stress from guilt will not improve anyone's health.

Further Information

• *Pregnancy, Children, and the Vegan Diet* by Michael Klaper, Gentle World Books, Maui, HI, 1987.

• *Simply Vegan* by Debra Wasserman, Vegetarian Research Group, Baltimore, MD, 1991.

• *Vegan Cookbook* by Alan Wakeman and Gordon Baskerville, Faber & Faber, Winchester, MA, 1986

• *Vegan Nutrition: A Survey of Research* by Gill Langley, The Vegan Society, London, England, 1990.

Personal Experiences
Susanna Rosenbaum

When I decided to have a fourth child, I was feeling great on a fairly low-fat, almost vegan diet, so I decided not to change. I was nursing a toddler once again, but he weaned during my pregnancy. I was extremely busy and active during my pregnancy and had a great deal of trouble gaining weight at all. I didn't gain an ounce until I was already five months pregnant. I attempted to add more fat and dairy products to my diet, but I could not tolerate them and had trouble with indigestion and constipation. I was not worried about my health nor was my midwife. My doctor was less sure. In the end, I gained only 20 pounds and my baby was small (six pounds, nine ounces) but in perfect health. He is now four months old: a big and fat baby who weighs about 18 pounds.

WEIGHT GAIN

During a healthy pregnancy, most women gain 25 to 30 pounds. During the first half of pregnancy, this is a direct shoring-up of the mother's nutritional reserves, with the largest gain an increase in total amount of maternal blood. A pregnant woman's breasts begin to fill out to be ready to produce and carry the milk the baby will need after birth.

In the second half of pregnancy, weight gain is primarily due to the growing size of the baby, as it approaches its birth weight, ideally 6 to 7 pounds. Weight gain throughout pregnancy is a positive sign, because it indicates that enough energy and nutrient intake is available for the baby to grow normally.

Ideal weight gain depends on your weight before pregnancy. A good rule of thumb is that if you are more than 10 percent underweight for your height before pregnancy, you should make an effort to gain that difference before you conceive, or at least add it to the total amount you should

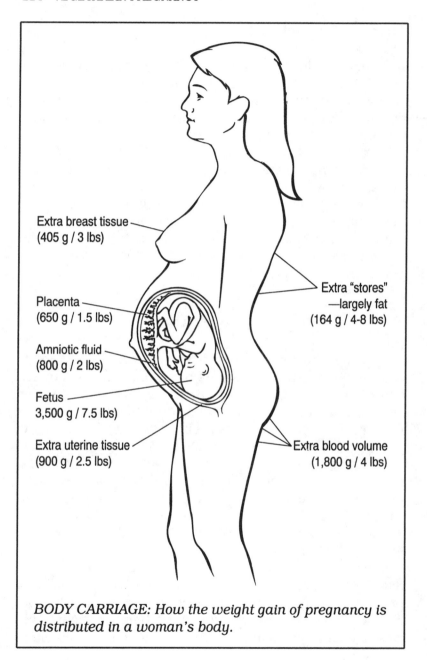

Extra breast tissue
(405 g / 3 lbs)

Placenta
(650 g / 1.5 lbs)

Amniotic fluid
(800 g / 2 lbs)

Fetus
3,500 g / 7.5 lbs)

Extra uterine tissue
(900 g / 2.5 lbs)

Extra "stores"
—largely fat
(164 g / 4-8 lbs)

Extra blood volume
(1,800 g / 4 lbs)

BODY CARRIAGE: How the weight gain of pregnancy is distributed in a woman's body.

ideally be expected to gain before the baby is born. If you are more than 20 percent overweight for your height, you should make an effort to lose a little weight before conception, since dieting is not a good idea during pregnancy.

Weight is a relative and a subjective issue when it comes to setting ideals, averages or norms. To say someone weighs 60 pounds is meaningless unless you know her age, at least. But saying someone weighs 120 pounds is not clarified by age alone: height is what is needed next. Weight depending upon height turns out to be a very useful way to look at large populations of people. It is so useful, in fact, that health and life insurance companies are able to use it to determine the actuarial odds and therefore increase their profits.

In determining maternal nutritional standards, the Subcommittee on Nutritional Status and Weight Gain During Pregnancy (appointed by the Institute of Medicine to prepare a report for the U.S. Department of Health and Human Services) found BMI, or body mass index (weight in pounds ÷ height in inches squared x 100), to be a better indicator of health than weight alone. The subcommittee agreed to the following definitions when assessing pre-pregnancy weight:

Underweight	Normal weight	Overweight	Obese
<2.8 BMI	2.8-3.7 BMI	3.7-4.1 BMI	>4.1 BMI

Are you underweight?

It is true that few vegetarians are extremely heavy, because the high fiber in their diet as well as the likely healthier balance of foods eaten tend to maintain a level of weight appropriate to body build. Being underweight is sometimes even considered a symbol of health in a meat- and fat-laden culture.

But when you are pregnant, being underweight is not so positive. Underweight mothers tend to have underweight babies, and low-birth-weight babies are more at risk for learning disabilities and other problems of early childhood.

Pre-pregnancy weight (in relationship to height) is important in assessing a mother's health. Before pregnancy, if a woman is more than 10 percent under the average weight for her height, she is considered *malnourished*. This is often commonly corrected by the larger-than-average appetite increase in early to middle pregnancy. (See "Digestion" and "Nausea/Morning Sickness") Since the baby does not put on substantial weight until the second half of pregnancy, these early months often are a natural way the mother's body compensates for being "underweight" before.

The rate of weight gain during pregnancy is also used to measure fetal health and development. If the rate of weight gain during pregnancy is insufficient, the mother is considered *undernourished*. This means that a wide variety of nutrients are not available to the mother or baby through daily diet, particularly those which provide energy: carbohydrates and proteins.

Fetal development, like human development, is unique but certain patterns have been observed. In a *New York Times* article (November 20, 1991), nutritionist Jane Brody reported that the failure of women to gain enough weight in the first and second trimesters of pregnancy is a major cause of their babies' low birth weight.

Her article reviewed a study of over 2,000 newborns researched by Dr. Theresa O. Scholl, an associate professor of obstetrics and gynecology at the School of Osteopathic Medicine at the University of Medicine and Dentistry in Newark, New Jersey. Although a link between overall pregnancy gain and birth weight had been discovered before, Scholl is one of the first doctors to study birth weight in the individual trimesters.

Dr. Scholl found that women who did not gain enough weight in the second trimester were likely to have low-birth-weight babies. Rather than a range of desirable weight gain of 24 to 30 pounds during the entire span of pregnancy, Scholl stressed the need for a 9- to 10-pound gain in the second trimester, with an even greater weight gain for pregnant teenage girls who are themselves still growing.

In the research world, the vegan diet is often cited as requiring additional care in the area of weight gain during pregnancy. Since the vegan diet is low in rich foods, it is necessary to eat greater quantities of other foods to obtain sufficient energy (carbohydrates and protein). A pregnant vegan needs to eat lots of pasta, cereals, breads and bananas if she has any problems gaining enough weight during pregnancy. (See "Vegan Pregnancy")

For a pregnant woman, appetite and stomach space are often at variance, particularly in the last few months when the baby is pushing on all parts of the digestive system. This may be of particular concern to any pregnant woman who eats a low-fat diet. Eating smaller meals more frequently— adding three more meals to the day instead of doubling the size of your three regular meals—is a good way to eat more without stuffing your stomach every time. Having less to digest will also speed the digestive process and you will probably be a lot more comfortable before and after meals.

Another way to increase weight gain is to reduce strenuous exercise (from aerobics to serious gardening). Walk rather than jog, swim rather than play volleyball. (See "Exercise") Don't become too sedentary, though, since regular movement is necessary for good digestion and the efficient working of all natural body systems.

Are you overweight?

Although the stereotype would imply otherwise, it is perfectly easy to gain weight on a vegetarian diet, primarily one that contains milk and dairy products. All animal foods are high in fats. When dairy products are added to rich carbohydrates such as cakes, cookies and breads, a mother can find herself putting on weight that is hard to take off.

Being slightly overweight is not harmful to a pregnancy. A woman has to be more than 20 percent over the norm (height for age) to be considered overweight, whereas only 10 percent under the norm is considered underweight.

If you are more than 30 percent overweight for your height and body type, you should try to get closer to your ideal weight by three months before conception. It is not easy on the body to lose weight, because often it is deprived of the required amounts of nutrients. A carbohydrate-free diet, for example, will accelerate the breakdown of tissue protein, which would be quite a deterrent to a developing fetus even if it does help an adult lose weight.

The Recommended Dietary Allowance for carbohydrates is related to the RDA for energy, which is about 2,200 calories/day. You can reduce your calories if they are above the RDA, but do not reduce them below the RDA, particularly once you are pregnant. Instead, when you become pregnant, 2,500 calories/day are recommended. Fats have nine calories per gram, almost twice the amount of protein (four calories per gram) or carbohydrates (also about four calories per gram).

Caloric requirements depend upon your activity level and weight. Naturally, the more active you are, the more energy (and calories) you need. To find out if you are getting enough calories, use the following formula:

Ideal Weight (for your height) x 12 (sedentary)
x 15 (moderately active)
x 22 (very active)

For example, if your ideal weight is 125, you need:

125 x 12 = 1,500 calories/day (sedentary)
125 x 15 = 1,875 calories/day (moderately active)
125 x 22 = 2,750 calories/day (very active)

The RDA of 2,200 assumes moderate activity and average adult female (ideal) weight/height. An additional 300 calories/day are recommended during pregnancy despite the mother's weight or height. This, however, is to be adjusted in the context of activity level and actual weight gain during pregnancy. A healthy diet sufficient in calories will produce a baby with normal or above-normal birth weight.

What's wrong with low birth weight?

When birth weight is low, the newborn's risk of health complications is higher. Low birth weight may cause learning disabilities which often do not become obvious until the child starts school. A greater vulnerability to infection and disease has been observed in low-birth-weight babies.

In cases of extremely low birth weight, fetal retardation may have occurred on one of two levels. The body may be smaller than average, but the head remains within the normal circumference range, indicating that normal mental development is likely. If the baby eats a lot after birth, natural growth mechanisms may compensate for earlier shortages and a baby can grow to normal size.

If birth weight is below 2,500 grams (5 pounds, 8 ounces), the baby's head circumference is likely to be smaller as well, indicating a higher chance of mental retardation. The body and skeleton seem to be affected first by lack of nutrition, with the brain continuing to grow at a normal rate. Only when the body and skeleton are extremely undernourished will the growth of the brain also be affected.

There seems to be a limit on the growth of babies. Normal-to-above-normal birth weights are found in babies of women whose weight near term is at least 120 percent of their pre-pregnancy weight, with 40 weeks' gestation. Pregnancy weights that exceed 120 percent do not result in any further increase in the size of the baby. If you weigh 125 pounds before pregnancy, you have the best chances for a healthy baby if you weigh at least 120 percent of that, or 150 pounds, when you go into labor. If you weigh more than that, you probably won't have a larger child, but if you weigh much less, you are putting your baby at risk.

Whether you are overweight or underweight, remember that a healthy diet is the most reliable way to have a healthy baby. A vegetarian diet with sufficient calories is the healthiest diet around.

Further Information

• "Impact of the Higgins Nutrition Intervention Program on birth weight: a within-mother analysis" by A.C. Higgins *et al., Journal of the American Dietetic Association,* 1989, 89: 1097-1103.

• *Nutrition During Pregnancy, Part I: Weight Gain* by The Institute of Medicine, National Academy Press, Washington, DC, 1990.

• *Nutrition in Pregnancy and Lactation, Fourth Edition* by Bonnie Worthington-Roberts and Sue Rodwell, eds., Mosby Publishing, St. Louis, MO, 1989.

• "Weight gain and pregnancy outcome in underweight and normal weight women" by Mary C. Mitchell and Edith Lerner, *Journal of the American Dietetic Association,* 1989, 89:634-641.

YOGA

Yoga is a gentle and timed-honored form of exercise that can keep your body healthy and relaxed without straining or bouncing, both of which are discouraged during pregnancy. Since I had studied and taught beginning yoga in college, I felt comfortable doing some yoga exercise on my own at home, with my husband joining me in the evenings. I started the yoga during the third month of my pregnancy and continued most of these exercises throughout. The following yoga positions are recommended for pregnant women and felt particularly good.

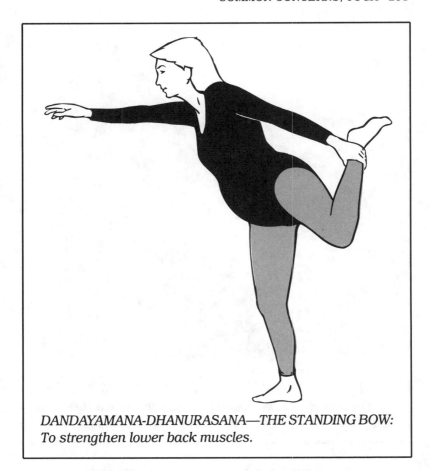

DANDAYAMANA-DHANURASANA—THE STANDING BOW:
To strengthen lower back muscles.

Dandayamana-dhanurasana (the standing bow pose)

• This position strengthens the muscles in the lower back, helping to prevent and relieve a common kind of backache during pregnancy. Your lower legs may get warmer after doing this exercise, because it helps with blood circulation as well. Balance on your right leg, leaning forward. Reach out with your right arm while reaching back with your left hand to clasp your left ankle. Move gently into position, and hold for eight to ten seconds, continuing to breathe slowly and steadily. Repeat, on the other leg. Do each side three times.

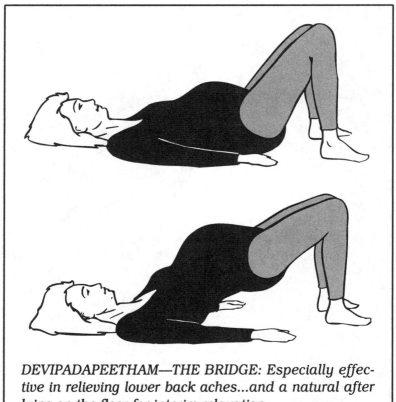

DEVIPADAPEETHAM—THE BRIDGE: Especially effective in relieving lower back aches...and a natural after lying on the floor for interim relaxation.

Interim relaxation (very important!)

• When you have completed any exercise, lie down on your back on a mat or other firm (but not too hard) surface, with your knees bent. Take five deep slow breaths, counting to three as you breathe in and counting to five as you breathe out.

Devipadapeetham (the bridge)

• This position is especially effective in relieving lower backaches and follows naturally when you are lying on the floor between exercises. Lie on your back with your knees

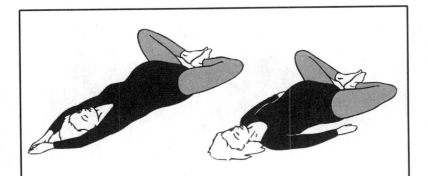

SUPTA-KONASANA—THIGH STRETCH: Helps to build endurance and strengthen pelvic muscles.

bent. Arch your back off the floor and inhale, while counting to five. Exhale to the count of five in place (with back arched as a bridge, arms on the floor for support) and then inhale to the count of five as you lower your back slowly to the floor. Exhale while counting to five, relaxing your back muscles. Repeat three times. Follow with the interim relaxation.

Supta-konasana (thigh stretch)

• Starting this asana (yoga position) during the first trimester will build strength and endurance. But it's important to continue practicing it during the last two months of pregnancy since it strengthens the pelvic floor muscles used in giving birth, by stretching pelvic joints, perineal and inner thigh muscles. Lie on your back with your feet together a few inches away from your buttocks. Relax your legs to either side without forcing them—do not stretch to the point of discomfort at any time. Breathing to a count of five, lift your clasped hands over your head and lay them on the ground above your head. Hold your breath for a count of three and lower your clasped hands to your abdomen while

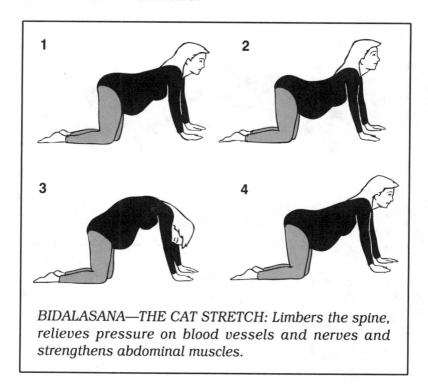

BIDALASANA—THE CAT STRETCH: Limbers the spine, relieves pressure on blood vessels and nerves and strengthens abdominal muscles.

exhaling and counting to five. Repeat three times and then relax in the interim relaxation position (see above).

Bidalasana (cat stretch)

• This position simulates the stretching of a cat as it gets up from a nap. It allows the abdominal organs to hang from the posterior abdominal wall, relieving the pressure on blood vessels and nerves that usually results from the force of gravity. The asana also limbers the spine, lower pelvis and hips while strengthening the abdominal muscles. It can be found in almost every book on exercise during pregnancy. Move to a count of five from a starting position on your hands and knees. Arch your back upwards and then downwards, holding each position for a count of three. After the second

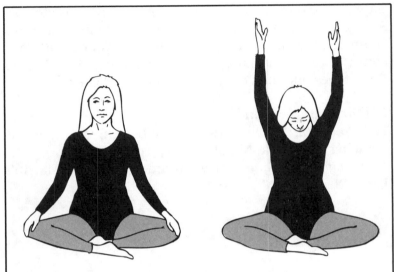

BADDHA-KONASANA—THE BOUND ANGLE: Strengthens pelvic and inner thigh muscles, and soothes indigestion.

upward arch of the back, extend the left leg back and then bring it back down slowly. Do another series of up and down stretches at the back and then extend the right leg. One important thing to remember is to breathe to the count of five with each movement, and to the count of three in between movements, holding each arch or leg extension. Repeat with each leg extension three times.

Baddha-konasana (bound angle pose)

• This position is another version of the Supta-konasana, done in a sitting position rather than lying down. It strengthens your pelvic joints, perineal and inner thigh muscles as it increases circulation to the breasts and strengthens the pectoral muscles which support them. The asana elevates the diaphragm and rib cage, allowing more room in the abdomen. This will help to relieve heartburn and indigestion.

Sit with the bottoms of your feet together and close to you. Rest your chin in the notch of your collarbone. Inhale to a count of five while raising your arms. Hold your breath for a count of three and lower them to a count of five. Repeat three times and then do the interim relaxation exercise.

Further Information
  • *Yoga During Pregnancy* by Vibeke Berg, Simon & Schuster, New York, NY, 1983.
  • *Yoga for Pregnancy* by Sandra Jordan, St. Martin's Press, New York, NY, 1988.

Chapter Four

Understanding Nutrients

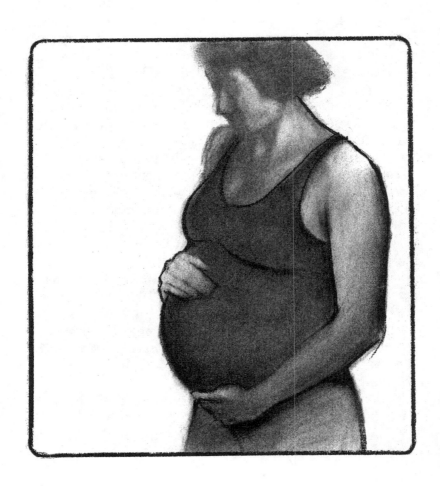

To answer specific questions which arise about individual nutrients, this section of *Vegetarian Pregnancy* will serve as a resource. The government's RDAs for pregnant women are listed for each nutrient, along with its known effects on gestation and possible problems stemming from any deficiencies or excesses during this time. The way each nutrient interacts with others is delineated as well, because a diet is never composed of isolated components.

A list of the foods which provide each nutrient is given at the end of each entry. In addition, when direct connections are known to exist, the nutrients are cross-referenced with Chapter Three, "Common Concerns."

The amount of information available on nutrition is tremendous, but I will list here a few important general reference works which I rely upon frequently. A complete bibliography can be found in the back of the book.

- *Nutrition Almanac* by Nutrition Search, Inc, McGraw-Hill, New York, NY, 1992.
- *Nutrition and Metabolism in Pregnancy* by Pedro Rosso, Oxford University Press, New York, NY, 1990.
- *Nutrition During Pregnancy* by The Institute of Medicine, National Academy Press, Washington, DC, 1990.
- *Recommended Dietary Allowances, 10th Edition* by The National Research Council, National Academy Press, Washington, DC 1989.
- *Transition to Vegetarianism* by Rudolph Ballentine, Himalayan International Institute, Honesdale, PA, 1987.
- *Vegan Nutrition: A Survey of Research* by Gill Langley, Vegan Society, London, England, 1988.

The following information is provided for each nutrient: the RDA, the need for supplementation, the effects of the nutrient on the mother and developing child, the effects of either a deficiency or an overdose of the nutrient, interactions with other nutrients, and good natural food sources. The nutrients discussed are grouped in three categories:

BIOTIN

RDA: 100 to 200 μg/day (no additional RDA for pregnancy)

Supplementation: No additional requirement for biotin during pregnancy. Biotin is not included in most vitamin supplements.

During Pregnancy: Biotin is a water-soluble vitamin that contains sulfur. It is synthesized in the lower gastrointestinal tract and available in trace amounts in all animal and plant tissue. Blood biotin levels decrease during pregnancy and continue to fall throughout gestation. However, no changes in birth weight or newborn health have been reported as a result of biotin in the diet.

Deficiency: A deficiency can be produced clinically by an excessive ingestion of raw egg whites, which binds biotin and prevents its absorption. (Cooking the egg white deactivates the binding element.)

Overdose: No known toxic effects.

Interactions: Antibiotics interfere with the production of the intestinal bacteria needed to synthesize biotin.

Sources: Biotin is found in whole grains, beans, brewer's yeast, mushrooms, cauliflower, dark green vegetables and chocolate.

CALCIUM

RDA: 1,200 mg/day (up from 800 mg for non-pregnant women over 25). Add 400 mg/day (total of 1,600 mg daily) if under 25 years of age.

Supplementation: If you have a low calcium intake, increase the level through calcium-rich foods, or less preferably, through a supplement. Since additional calcium is needed during pregnancy, many doctors frequently recommend a multi-vitamin/mineral supplement that includes calcium. Natural derivatives of calcium which are easy to absorb are calcium gluconate and calcium lactate. It is available but less useful as bone meal (an animal product). For best absorption, take a supplement with a low-protein meal.

Calcium supplementation has been used effectively to lower blood pressure, decrease premature births, and decrease the incidence of pre-eclampsia when symptoms indicate these problems are present during pregnancy. However, self-medication with calcium for these concerns is possibly dangerous, since calcium increases smooth-muscle activity and, if taken in excess, could induce uterine contractions, starting an early labor.

During Pregnancy: Calcium is the most abundant mineral in the body; 99 percent of it is found in the bones and teeth. Calcium assists in building and maintaining bones, teeth, healthy blood and proper blood clotting. It aids in the utilization of iron and helps regulate the passage of nutrients in and out of cell walls. It can ease insomnia. The National Research Council does not recommend routine lab testing for calcium status in pregnant women.

During pregnancy, calcium metabolism undergoes drastic changes, including increased intestinal absorption, greater calcium retention and elevation in the plasma concentration of aparathyroid hormone. Between 20 to 40 weeks of gestation, the average fetus accumulates 28 grams of calcium daily. The placenta itself synthesizes something called "1,25(OH)2D" which assists in increasing calcium absorption by the intestines. This may be a factor contributing to the infrequency of calcium deficiency noted in pregnant women.

Deficiency: Muscle spasms and cramps, numbness and tingling in the arms and legs are the first signs of a calcium deficiency. Although a direct connection has not been established, leg cramps, which are common in pregnancy, can sometimes (but not always) be relieved by adding more calcium to your diet.

Overdose: Excesses may cause hypercalcemia or excessive calcification of the bones and other tissues (such as the liver), may interfere with nervous and muscular system functioning, and reduce the body's absorption of zinc, particularly important in pregnancy. (See "Zinc")

Interactions: The ratio of calcium to phosphorus in bones is 2.5 to 1; the body must have a proper phosphorus/calcium balance available to maintain bone strength. Calcium must also be in the presence of magnesium, vitamins A, C, D, and possibly E to be used by the body in developing and maintaining healthy bones and teeth. Excessive stress, excitement or depression can inhibit or interfere with calcium absorption.

Calcium utilization in humans is profoundly affected by the level of dietary intake, according to a report by Michael B. Zemel in the *American Journal of Clinical Nutrition.* The more protein that is eaten, the more calcium is excreted from the body. A soy-based diet provides an excellent low calcium/protein balance.

Large amounts of phytic acid, the fiber in cereals and grains, can bind calcium and prevent its absorption. Bran is particularly high in phytic acid, so its use as a laxative may have some negative side effects, particularly during pregnancy. Leavening increases the absorbability of calcium from baked goods.

Oxalic acid, found in green leafy vegetables, interferes with calcium absorption. Spinach and chard contain especially high levels of oxalic acid. However, if rice is eaten with these vegetables, it prevents this interference and allows for good calcium absorption from these otherwise nutritious vegetables. Grains other than rice have not been found to be as effective in doing this. Other calcium-rich leafy vegetables such as kale, collards and mustard greens have much lower oxalic acid levels naturally, and do not need rice for proper absorption.

Sources: Calcium is found in dark green vegetables (kale, collard greens, broccoli, mustard greens, spinach, chard), blackstrap molasses, seaweeds, sesame seeds, tahini and dairy products.

CARBOHYDRATES

RDA: Energy requirements are filled by carbohydrates, proteins, fats and oils. Carbohydrate requirements are expressed in kilocalories (kcal) and the number of calories you require depends on your weight. The recommended energy intake *before* pregnancy is 1,900 to 2,200 kcal/day for most women (women weighing less need fewer kcal, women weighing more require more to maintain weight). Pregnancy increases the need by 300 kcal/day, regardless of pre-conception weight.

Supplementation: If the stereotype of the underweight vegetarian applies to you, you should eat more (healthy) carbohydrates especially to increase your weight before pregnancy. If mothers are underweight at conception, their babies are more likely to be born underweight which increases infants' health risks during the first year of life. (See "Common Concerns: Weight Gain") Carbohydrates are taken as a supplement in the form of more food, particularly whole grain breads and cereals.

During Pregnancy: Carbohydrates, proteins and fats, are the three food sources of energy, essential to life. Carbohydrates are necessary for the digestion and assimilation of other foods; they are used by the digestive system to regulate protein and fat metabolism.

Fats contain nine calories per gram, more than twice the amount than proteins or carbohydrates (four calories per gram). The RDA recommends that more than half of the human energy requirement be filled by carbohydrate rather than fat after infancy. For example, whole grain foods are a better source of carbohydrates than milk for an adult, while milk is more appropriate for an infant.

During pregnancy, a natural increase in appetite usually provides the incentive to consume the extra 300 kcal required daily for healthy fetal development. Carbohydrates are essential during this time to maintain maternal health and energy, as well as providing the basic fuel for new life. Carbohydrate metabolism undergoes several changes as a result of pregnancy: plasma glucose levels decline, basal and stimulated insulin secretion increases, and insulin-sensitive tissues develop some degree of resistance to the action of this hormone.

The two kinds of digestible carbohydrates in food are sugars (simple carbohydrates) and starches (complex carbohydrates). Cellulose is an indigestible carbohydrate that provides the bulk and fiber necessary to aid in cleaning of the digestive system and in elimination. Eating "healthy" carbohydrates (real foods) is the best way to add calories to your diet during pregnancy; "empty" carbohydrates (junk foods) just put on weight without increasing nutrient levels at all.

Deficiency: If you don't get enough carbohydrates, you are more likely to have a low-birth-weight baby (less than 5 pounds, 8 ounces, or 2,500 grams). Low birth weight frequently results in learning problems and other minor disabilities as well as an increased chance of health risks, especially during the first year of life. (See "Common Concerns: Weight Gain")

Overdose: Excessive carbohydrate intake slows down digestion and metabolism. This is likely to result in intestinal discomfort and unnecessary weight gain. An excessive number of calories may indicate or produce a nutritional imbalance. Higher carbohydrate intake increases the amount of calcium excreted in the urine. (Excess protein and sodium increases will also increase calcium excretion.)

Interactions: Individual carbohydrate requirements vary depending upon your activity and metabolism levels. If you are very physically active, you will need more carbohydrates than if you have a sedentary life. The type of carbohydrate you eat must be taken into account as well: processed foods such as white flour, white sugar and polished rice cause a relative vitamin B deficiency when eaten in excess.

Sources: The additional carbohydrate requirements of pregnancy can be met by a daily addition to your diet of a variety of foods, such as these: one blueberry muffin, one bagel, ¾ cup wheat germ cereal, one avocado, ten halves of dried peaches.

Sometimes it is necessary to substitute more complex carbohydrates with greater nutrient values (whole grain cereals and breads) for simpler carbohydrates with less or no nutrient value (many packaged snack foods).

CHLORIDES

RDA: No RDA has been set for chlorides.

Supplementation: Chlorides are so easily available that they do not require supplementation and are not included in vitamin or mineral supplements.

During Pregnancy: Chloride salts of sodium and potassium regulate the correct balance of acid and alkali (pH) in the blood and maintain pressure that causes fluids to pass in and out of cell membranes. Chlorides also work in digestion of protein and fibrous foods by stimulating the liver and helping to clean toxic waste from the body. Other than general body maintenance, the effects of chlorides on pregnancy are not specifically noted in any research.

Deficiency: It is extremely unlikely that you would get too little chloride in your diet, particularly if you use table salt (sodium chloride) at all. No deficiencies of this nutrient have been reported.

Overdose: Daily intake over 14 grams of salt is considered excessive and has been linked to high blood pressure in some people. (See SODIUM) Potassium chloride overdoses are highly unlikely and have not been observed.

Interactions: The presence of chlorides is essential to the proper functioning of sodium and potassium in the digestive process.

Sources: Table salt (sodium chloride), natural water.

CHOLINE

RDA: No RDA has been set for choline.

Supplementation: Since no RDA has been established for choline, it is rarely included in multiple vitamin/mineral supplements.

During Pregnancy: Choline is one of the B complex vitamins and a component of lecithin. The placenta both synthesizes choline and actively transports it from the mother to the fetus. The demand for choline-containing compounds is high during growth and development.

Deficiency: A deficiency of choline may contribute to liver damage in the presence of alcohol. Choline deficiency will result in fatty deposits in the liver, heart trouble and high blood pressure.

Overdose: Excessive dosages may reduce B_6 availability.

Interactions: Too little protein in the diet may cause a deficiency in choline.

Sources: Choline is found in wheat germ and brewer's yeast.

CHROMIUM

RDA: No RDA has been established, but a range of 50 to 200 µg/day is considered safe and adequate.

Supplementation: According to a summary of data by the Institute on Medicine, there is no research to indicate any need for additional chromium during pregnancy. This is especially true on a varied whole foods diet and less true on a diet high in processed foods. Most supplements do not include chromium.

During Pregnancy: Chromium is an essential mineral found in the blood, regulating blood sugar levels through assisting insulin to attach itself to the proper receptacles. It is hard to measure and analyze, but no symptoms of chromium deficiency have been seen in adults consuming 50 µg/day. Chromium picolinate is the easiest form of chromium to assimilate. Pregnant women may be particularly susceptible to chromium deficiency because of high fetal demand during development.

Deficiency: Even a slight deficiency of chromium can cause an insulin dysfunction. Chromium concentrations in human tissues naturally decline with age, except in the lungs where it accumulates. For this reason, older women who are pregnant should be especially conscious of their chromium intake. Chromium levels in foods may be particularly low in the United States, where soils have been depleted and foods refined.

Overdose: One is unlikely to get too much chromium through the diet alone. A 200 µg/day supplement has produced no adverse effects, but amounts above that level have not yet been established as safe.

Interactions: Refining of commercial foods results in a loss of up to 98 percent of chromium content, according to *Total Health* magazine. Chromium speeds up fat metabolism and may help to suppress appetite and cravings for sweets.

Sources: Good bio-availability has been found in whole wheat bread, whole grain cereals, brewer's yeast and wheat germ, but the chromium content of most foods has not been established yet.

COPPER

RDA: The RDA for copper is 1.5 to 3 mg daily. Copper retention is only about 40 percent of that ingested, and the RDA takes this factor into account when determining the amount that should be present in the diet.

Supplementation: Copper levels rarely fall during the first two trimesters, so supplementation seems unwarranted. During the third trimester, copper intake is usually lower than estimated copper requirements, but there is no evidence that fetal growth and development are jeopardized as a result. Therefore, no recommendation is generally made for prenatal copper supplementation.

During Pregnancy: Copper is a trace mineral necessary for proper bone formation and for the production of RNA. Plasma levels of copper increase during pregnancy, reaching 2 to 2.5 mg over non-pregnancy levels near term. Copper levels in maternal tissue decrease as plasma levels rise. By birth, the fetus contains about 14 mg of copper and the placenta an additional 6 mg. Copper is partially stored in the baby's liver for use during the first few months of life (copper in mother's milk is minimal.)

Deficiency: Copper deficiencies in the human diet are rare, although infants fed solely on cow's milk for extended periods of time during hospitalization developed symptoms of deficiency which included bone demineralization and anemia. Extreme maternal copper deficiency has been found to be the cause of infertility, spontaneous abortions and stillbirths as well as severe physical abnormalities.

Toxicity: Copper toxicity is rare, but has been observed in people ingesting more than 8 mg/day, which could result from using primarily copper pans, cups and bowls.

Interactions: Copper retention is lowered by a zinc supplementation of 20 mg or more a day. If supplementation seems appropriate, a 2 mg dosage should be taken if you are also taking a zinc supplement. (See "Zinc") This is a high enough dosage to compensate for reduced copper absorption due to the zinc.

Sources: Copper is available in legumes, nuts, seeds, whole grains and any plant foods grown in copper-rich soil. Ironically, copper is presently quite available in most diets due to copper-containing fungicides that have been sprayed on agricultural products. You may also get copper from your water supply if it's carried in copper plumbing.

ENERGY

RDA: An average of 2,500 kcal/day is recommended to meet the energy requirements of pregnancy, up 300 kcal/day over the recommendation for non-pregnant adult women. The RDA for energy is expressed as kilocalories per day of potential food energy that can be absorbed and utilized.

Supplementation: Eat more carbohydrates and balanced proteins if weight gain or rate of weight gain is not adequate. (See "Common Concerns: Weight Gain")

During Pregnancy: Additional energy is needed during pregnancy because a baby takes a lot of energy to grow. A woman's basal metabolism increases during pregnancy and appetite increases as well, providing a natural adjustment in the body to the increased energy demand. The amount of energy used during pregnancy is estimated to be about 80,000 kcal. Sufficient energy intake is measured by the rate of weight gain during pregnancy

Low energy before pregnancy (malnutrition) and too little energy during pregnancy (gestational undernutrition) are two ways that body reserves can be depleted. Unless a woman begins pregnancy underweight, she won't need to increase her energy "charging" during the first trimester. "Underweight" is defined as more than 10 percent below the norms for one's height/weight ratio. If you are underweight before pregnancy, it will be helpful to your baby's growth and development to increase your intake of healthy foods right away, to bring yourself within normal range. Energy needs are highest during the second trimester, and a little lower in the third trimester, when energy is usually conserved by a lower rate of activity as the woman's pregnant weight slows her down.

Deficiency: Too little energy (kilocalories) can result in a lower-birth-weight baby who will be at higher risk for learning disabilities and infections. (See "Common Concerns: Weight Gain") An intake below 1,900 kcal/day is considered low in calories. Fasting may increase the chance of an early labor. Evidence indicates that pregnant women are more likely to have an energy deficiency in the diet than a protein deficiency.

Toxicity: If she takes in too many calories, a woman will gain too much weight, resulting in a heavier load on all body systems. Current wisdom suggests that gaining a little too much weight during pregnancy is preferable to gaining too little in terms of the health of the mother and baby, before and after birth. If you are thin before getting pregnant, your body will try to make up the missing amount and so a weight gain slightly above average is normal.

Interactions: Movement and exercise affect the efficiency of the body in digesting and utilizing nutrients. Some exercise is good for you and will help digestion and effective use of energy. Too much exercise, stress and tension will deplete your energy. (See "Common Concerns: Exercise")

Sources: Carbohydrates, fats and proteins are the sources of energy in the diet. All foods provide some energy.

FATS

RDA: There is no RDA for fats, but they should not exceed 25 to 30 percent of caloric intake. Less than 10 percent of calories should be provided from saturated fatty acids and at least 2 percent of calories should be linoleic acid.

Supplementation: Essential fatty acids, crucial to optimal digestion, may be missing in most American diets. Although these are available in oils, nuts, seeds and seafood, supplements are available. However, supplements of eicosapentaenoic acid (EPA) and docosahexaenoic acid (DHA) can reduce natural blood-clotting abilities as well as increase blood sugar levels with concurrent declines in insulin production. It is wise to avoid these supplements during pregnancy.

During Pregnancy: Fats are the most concentrated form of energy from food, with one gram of fat yielding about nine calories. (See "Energy") Fats slow down the stomach's secretions of hydrochloric acid, keeping nutrients in the digestive system longer, increasing absorption time. In this way, fats in a meal create the sensation of fullness after a meal. A meal of animal foods will take longer to digest than a meal of plant foods only. Since feeling too full is common for pregnant women, particularly during the last trimester, a vegetarian diet is likely to be a lot more comfortable than a meat-centered one during pregnancy.

There are two kinds of fatty acids: saturated (hard at room temperature, primarily from animal sources, except for coconut) and unsaturated (usually liquid at room temperature, primarily from plant sources.) Three fatty acids are considered essential, with one, linoleic acid, being the precursor to the other two, arachidonic acid and linolenic acid). The essential fatty acids are necessary for normal growth and healthy blood, arteries and nerves. They keep the skin and other tissues youthful and healthy by preventing dryness and scaliness. Essential fatty acids are necessary for the transport and breakdown of cholesterol as well as for the production of prostaglandins, which are regulators of the cardiovascular, reproductive and immune systems.

Research suggests that sufficient maternal weight gain, including some maternal fat storage, is needed to ensure that the size of the newborn is optimal and that sufficient energy for lactation is available after birth. A woman who gains 25 pounds during pregnancy uses about $5\frac{1}{2}$ pounds of fat during the first few months of breast-feeding; fat stores can theoretically provide about 100 to 150 kcal/day for the first six months of lactation.

Deficiency: If essential fatty acids are missing from the diet, skin disorders may result. If deficiency is severe, growth will be retarded in the fetus.

Toxicity: Since fats take a long time to digest, too high a level in the diet may result in abnormal weight gain and obesity as well as a continued feeling of indigestion. (See "Common Concerns: Weight Gain")

Interactions: Adequate dietary fat is necessary for proper absorption of vitamins A, E, D and K.

Sources: Linoleic acid is found in vegetable oils such as corn, safflower and soybean. Oils made from canola, flax and hemp seed are particularly good plant sources. Most nuts, seeds and seafood also contain linoleic acid. Cold-water seafood provides the other two essential fatty acids.

FLUORIDES

RDA: The estimated range of safe and adequate intake of fluorides is 1.5 to 4.0 mg/day, or 1 part per million, or 1 mg/liter of liquid.

Supplementation: A report on maternal nutrition by the Institute of Medicine concludes that there is not enough evidence to warrant routine fluoride supplementation during pregnancy as a way to strengthen the baby's developing teeth. A high level of water fluoridation has been implicated in an increased chance of Down's syndrome, so check the fluoride content of your water level before taking fluoride supplements! (Call your local health department for details about the public water supply in your area.)

During Pregnancy: Fluorine is a trace element found in almost every tissue in the body, in compounds called fluorides. The two main fluoride salts in the diet are: sodium fluoride, which is added to drinking water, and calcium fluoride, found naturally in foods. The absorption of fluoride from sodium fluoride in water is estimated to be 100 percent. Fluorine deficiencies are rare in the United States, because public water is commonly fluoridated to a concentration between 0.7 and 1.2 mg/liter. (The Food and Nutrition Board recommends fluoridation of public water if the natural concentration of fluorides is below 0.7 mg/liter.)

Evidence indicates that supplementing a child's diet with fluorides protects teeth during the first two to four years of life. Other studies have found that supplementation during pregnancy is positively correlated with fewer dental caries after birth in the child. However, no direct evidence shows that fluorides protect teeth before they erupt.

Deficiency: If too little fluoride is available, tooth decay becomes more likely and bones may be softened.

Toxicity: More than 2 mg/liter of fluorides (twice the recommended level) is considered toxic, with tooth mottling one of the first signs of excess fluorides. Excessive fluorides can destroy the enzyme phosphatase which assists in the metabolism of vitamins. Excess fluoride can also inhibit the activities of other important enzymes and appears to be especially "antagonistic" toward brain tissues. With daily exposures of over 20 mg, chronic toxicity affects bone health, kidney, muscle and nerve functions.

Interactions: Calcium may interfere with fluoride absorption and is an antidote for fluoride poisoning.

Sources: Teas! In countries such as England, where tea drinking is common, tea may be a primary source of fluorides in the diet of adults, up to 1.3 mg of the average daily intake of 1.8 mg. Other sources are more commercial: fluoride toothpastes and fluoride pills, available from most dentists.

FOLIC ACID
Other names for this nutrient are folacin and folate.

RDA: During pregnancy, the RDA for folate is set at 400 µg/day, an increase of 220 µg/day—more than twice as much as is recommended before pregnancy. The additional folate is needed to build and maintain the maternal folate stores which are used to support rapidly growing tissues in the mother and the fetus, as well as the placenta. This RDA level is based on the fact that only about 50 percent of food folate is absorbed by the human body.

Supplementation: The recommendation of 400 µg/day can be met by a well-selected diet without food fortification or oral supplementation. Recent reports by the United States Public Health Service found folic acid to be so essential in the prevention of birth defects that folic acid supplements were recommended to all women of child-bearing age. Other reports argue against routine supplementation, but "modest" supplementation is often recommended to pregnant women who smoke, drink and/or do not eat a well-balanced diet. Folic acid may also be recommended for pregnant adolescents or women carrying more than one child. Folic acid deficiency is a particular risk for pregnant women who do not include many fresh greens in their daily diet. In a balanced vegetarian diet, leafy greens are standard fare, so most pregnant vegetarians have a natural advantage.

During Pregnancy: Pregnancy does not affect the efficiency of folic acid absorption, so folic acid requirements jump dramatically during pregnancy due to increased blood supply in the mother and the growth of the fetus. Folic acid is involved in the production of nucleic acid which is essential for the processes of growth and reproduction of all tissues in the body. Folic acid increases the appetite and helps the liver work efficiently. Folate and folacin are generic terms for compounds that have nutritional properties and chemical structures similar to those of folic acid.

Deficiency: Instances of too little folic acid during pregnancy have been well-studied and well-documented. The World Health Organization found that one-third to one-half of pregnant women have folic acid deficiencies during their third trimester. If folic acid is not sufficiently available to the fetus, it can result in deformities such as cleft palate, neural defects and brain damage before birth. Folic acid deficiencies have been linked to low birth weight, slower development and learning disabilities after birth as well.

Since folic acid is crucial in even the first weeks of pregnancy, make sure that you increase your folic acid intake (through dietary sources if possible) before conception. The first trimester of pregnancy involves a higher risk of folic acid deficiency than for any other nutrient important to healthy development. The third trimester, when pregnancy requires a huge increase in the baby's hemoglobin, is also a risk period for folic acid deficiency, since daily supply must be increased to meet the demand.

Toxicity: No known toxicity, although an excessive intake may cover up a B_{12} deficiency. (See "Vitamin B_{12}: Deficiency" and "Common Concerns: Anemia/Iron Deficiency") Folic acid is readily excreted in the urine; it is water soluble, so toxicity is unlikely to occur. However, doses more than 100 times the RDA have been reported to cause convulsions in some epileptics.

Interactions: Up to 50 percent of food folate may be destroyed by food processing and storage. Heat, oxidation and light destroy the nutritional value of the folic acid molecule. Sulfa drugs interfere with the intestinal bacteria that manufacture folic acid. Oral contraceptives, alcohol and antibiotics such as aminopterin and streptomycin can also interfere with and destroy folic acid. Stress and disease increase the body's need for this nutrient. Folic acid is part of the vitamin B complex, and works best when combined with other B vitamins and vitamin C.

Sources: Folic acid intake is vital to a healthy pregnancy, but it can usually be obtained from the diet (green vegetables such as broccoli, spinach and other dark leafy vegetables as well as brewer's yeast are especially recommended). Significant amounts of folic acid are also found in whole or fortified breads and cereals, dried peas and beans, and fruits of all kinds. Herbal sources include watercress, parsley, chicory, and dandelion greens. Raw greens retain more folic acid than cooked ones.

INOSITOL

RDA: No RDA, or safe and adequate levels have been established by the National Research Council.

Supplementation: Because no RDA has been set for inositol, it is rarely found in a multi-vitamin supplement. If a supplement is deemed necessary, avoid inositol in its phosphate form since the phosphate ester of inositol inhibits zinc absorption. Always take supplemental inositol with other B vitamins since the B complex must be kept in balance.

During Pregnancy: Inositol is part of the B vitamin complex; the human body contains more inositol than any vitamin other than niacin. Inositol promotes the body's production of lecithin and is helpful in brain cell nutrition. About 7 percent of the inositol that is ingested is changed into glucose. The average daily consumption of inositol by adults in the United States is about one gram. Inositol has a soothing effect, may alleviate insomnia and gradually lower blood pressure, and is given to people with high serum copper and low serum zinc levels. Inositol has not been documented to have any affect uniquely related to pregnancy.

Deficiency: A deficiency of inositol can cause constipation, eczema, abnormalities of the eyes, high blood cholesterol levels, and hair loss in the mother. Effects of an inositol deficiency in a fetus have not been determined.

Toxicity: No known toxicity (although it doesn't seem to be well researched) but should never be taken in excess alone, just as with any other B vitamin.

Interactions: Caffeine can deplete the body's stores of inositol. Stress, lack of exercise and alcohol affect the B vitamin complex as a whole, reducing inositol levels as well as the other components of the B complex.

Sources: Large quantities of inositol are found in lecithin. One tablespoon of brewer's yeast contains 40 mg inositol. It is also available in unprocessed whole grains, citrus fruits and unrefined molasses.

IODINE

RDA: The RDA for iodine is 175 µg/day, up 25 µg/day from the pre-conception recommendation.

Supplementation: Most diets in the United States show no evidence of an iodine deficiency, probably due to the prevalence of iodized salt. Iodine deficiencies are more common in areas where iodized salt is not available, such as Africa, Asia and South America.

During Pregnancy: An essential micro-nutrient for all animals, iodine is converted into iodide inside the body. This trace element is best known for its importance to healthy functioning of the thyroid gland. Iodine is also involved in regulating energy production, promoting growth and development, and stimulating the rate of metabolism. Iodine may be a key micro-nutrient for healthy neurological development.

Deficiency: An iodine deficiency may result in deafness, stillbirth, spontaneous abortions and milder neurological impairments. Cretinism is a congenital disease characterized by physical and mental retardation in children born to mothers who have had an iodine deficiency during adolescence and pregnancy. Many of the symptoms of an iodine deficiency are reversible, but if conditions persist beyond childbirth or possibly early infancy, the mental and physical retardation will be permanent. A deficiency may be present in the fetus without clinical signs of deficiency (such as hypothyroidism) in the mother, but usually a deficiency can be detected in the mother first. An iodine deficiency should be corrected prior to conception to avoid damage to the fetus.

Toxicity: There is no known toxicity level for iodine obtained through foods. Medical doses can be toxic, interfering with the synthesis of thyroid hormones and resulting in goiter and thyrotoxicosis.

Interactions: Raw cabbage and nuts contain compounds which may interfere with iodine use in thyroid functioning.

Sources: If you avoid iodized table salt, make sure you have iodized sea salt, sea vegetables and mushrooms (often grown in iodized soil) in your diet to provide this essential nutrient.

IRON

RDA: The RDA for iron for pregnant women is 30 mg/day, double that of the non-pregnant adult female requirement, and *three* times that of a teenage girl's requirement.

Supplementation: Indiscriminate iron supplementation is not recommended for pregnant women, even though this is a common practice. In many cases, the supplemental iron dosage prescribed is too high, and it has been observed that too much iron can reduce levels of zinc in the blood. (See "Zinc") Iron supplements are hard on the digestive system, frequently causing constipation, which is a common problem for pregnant women anyway. (See "Common Concerns: Constipation") Ferrous sulfate is a commonly prescribed form of iron but it is very poorly absorbed (only 10 to 30 percent), and can be hard on the liver, kidneys and intestines during digestion. Iron supplements should generally be taken between meals with liquids other than milk, tea or coffee. Iron from food sources and herbal supplements are most preferable, having fewer side effects.

During Pregnancy: Red cell mass in the blood increases by 18 percent during pregnancy, requiring 300 to 500 mg of additional iron. The additional 283 mg of iron in a full-term fetus, and 75 mg more of iron contained in the placenta suggest a minimum extra iron requirement of almost 700 mg during pregnancy. These increased needs are met by mobilization of stored iron and increased intestinal iron absorption. This may represent a total of 3 to 6 mg of iron absorbed daily, up from 1 to 2 mg/day prior to conception. The cumulative difference may amount to 280 to 560 mg during the last half of pregnancy. The placenta has an upper limit to the amount of iron it can transfer to the fetus. Instead, the mother stores the excess iron until it can be used by the placenta.

Deficiency: Iron anemia during pregnancy is normal to a certain extent. As blood supplies in the mother and fetus increase, greater iron is needed to transfer the oxygen. (See "Common Concerns: Anemia") The mother's body copes with this in two ways: first, menstruation ceases, greatly decreasing the loss of iron-rich blood. Second, the rate of iron absorption increases by five percent during pregnancy. This increase is seen most clearly during the second trimester, particularly if an iron deficiency exists at that point.

Most American women enter pregnancy with low or depleted stores, so if your diet is not rich in iron already, pre-conception is a good time to increase your iron intake. A normal hemoglobin count is 12 to 16 grams per 100 milliliters of blood, or a density of 35 to 49 percent. A reading of under 12 grams or 35 percent is considered anemic. (See "Common Concerns: Anemia") Iron deficiency in the mother will result in reduced birth weight in the baby, with all the related problems that can bring. (See "Common Concerns: Weight Gain")

Toxicity: Too much iron will upset the utilization of several other nutrients, including zinc, manganese and copper, which are essential to a healthy pregnancy. Constipation is a common side effect of most iron supplements. Iron is one of the nutrients that can potentially exert toxic effects on the fetus. Recent reports in *The New York Times* suggest that too much iron in the diet can contribute to a variety of blood diseases in adults as well.

Interactions: Iron supplementation may interfere with zinc, copper and manganese absorption. Vitamin E inhibits the absorption of inorganic iron, and supplements for these two nutrients should be taken separately. (I was told to take an E supplement eight hours after the iron supplement.) Drinking tea also inhibits iron absorption. Vitamin C (fruit juices, fruits) enhance the absorption of iron.

Sources: Eating citrus or other vitamin C-rich foods along with iron-rich foods such as spinach or grains increases iron absorption. Cooking in iron cookware will dramatically increase the iron content of foods. Some kinds of soy products have iron that is more accessible than others, according to a report in the August 1991 *Vegetarian Times*. Lucy Moll reports that silken tofu, tempeh (fermented soybeans), natto (fermented whole soybeans) and miso raised iron levels higher than regular tofu, fermented tofu or soy flour. Silken tofu, which is not fermented, is low in calcium, an iron inhibitor. Herbal sources of iron include yellow dock root, parsley, nettles, dandelion root, kelp and amaranth greens.

In a study by Elaine R. Monsen in the *Journal of the American Dietetic Association*, vegetarian diets may naturally offer high iron availability, partly because of the higher ratio of foods rich in ascorbic acid that are likely to be found in the vegetarian diet. Vegetarians were more likely to have adequate hemoglobin and iron stores in their body than those who ate meat, fish or poultry as their primary protein source, according to her report.

The macrobiotic diet uses many foods that are less familiar, but includes some foods particularly high in iron. For example, miso soups, various seaweed dishes using hijiki, kombu, dulse and green nori flakes, adzuki bean dishes and roasted squash and pumpkin seeds are recommended by Michio and Aveline Kushi for their high iron content. (See "Common Concerns: Macrobiotic Pregnancy")

MAGNESIUM

RDA: The RDA for magnesium is 300 mg/day, up 20 mg from the recommendation for non-pregnancy.

Supplementation: Most people have a dietary deficiency of magnesium but display no obvious symptoms. In limited studies, supplementation was found to decrease the number of cases of fetal growth retardation and pre-eclampsia, but more research is needed to warrant routine magnesium supplementation for pregnant women. Magnesium can interfere with iron absorption so don't take both nutrients in the same supplement.

During Pregnancy: Magnesium, part of the green pigment of chlorophyll, activates more than 300 enzymes, including those necessary for metabolism of carbohydrates and amino acids. It is essential to the health of the nervous system and has been used successfully to control convulsions in pregnant women. Magnesium balances the stimulative effect of calcium, playing an important regulatory role during muscle use. It is very alkaline, acting like an antacid—magnesium can replace over-the-counter antacid compounds such as milk of magnesia. It is sometimes prescribed by doctors for women who are experiencing an unusual degree of nausea during pregnancy.

Magnesium levels normally rise during the onset of pregnancy and fall to base levels during the last trimester. In the presence of magnesium, the placenta can accumulate calcium for active transfer to the fetus. During the last two trimesters of pregnancy, the placenta transfers magnesium to the fetus at the rate of 6 mg/day.

Deficiency: No signs of magnesium deficiency have been observed in most U.S. diets even though average magnesium intake is lower than the RDA. However, magnesium has been used to treat diarrhea, vomiting, nervousness and kwashiorkor. Chronic magnesium deficiency is thought to be linked to coronary heart disease. Symptoms of a magnesium deficiency include muscle twitches, tremors, irregular heart rhythm, depression and disorientation. There is some indication that painful uterine contractions sometimes experienced at the end of a pregnancy result from a magnesium deficiency.

Toxicity: Supplements, rather than magnesium-rich foods, are the likely culprits in an overdose. Early signs of magnesium toxicity include nausea, vomiting and hypotension.

Interactions: Magnesium promotes absorption and metabolism of many important nutrients, including calcium, phosphorus, sodium, potassium, the B vitamins, C and E. The balance between magnesium and calcium is particularly important—if calcium intake is high, magnesium intake also needs to be high. High blood cholesterol levels and/or high protein consumption can also increase the body's need for magnesium. Magnesium is refined out of foods during processing and cooking. Vitamin D must be present for magnesium to work.

Sources: Magnesium is found in all unprocessed plant foods, especially grains and vegetables. More than 80 percent of magnesium is lost when grains are refined. Green vegetables are especially rich in magnesium; bananas are one of the only fruits containing a significant amount.

MANGANESE

RDA: 2 to 5 mg/day of manganese is recommended for adults, with no additional manganese required for a healthy pregnancy.

Supplementation: Supplementation is not needed during pregnancy. An occasional intake of 10 mg/day by adults is considered safe by the National Research Council, but recommended intake levels are much lower.

During Pregnancy: Manganese is a trace mineral necessary for normal skeletal development, the formation of blood, and nourishment of the nerves and brain. Internal homeostatic controls and easy availability in the food supply seem to insure a constancy in the level stored and available during pregnancy. Manganese is a crucial element in the production of milk during nursing.

Deficiency: Because manganese is so widely available in plant foods relative to human requirements, a deficiency is unlikely. Manganese deficiencies observed in institutionalized populations (where fresh plant foods in the diet are minimal) have been associated with reduced glucose tolerance, dizziness, ear noises, loss of hearing and muscle coordination failure in adults. Manganese deficiencies have also been linked with infertility, growth retardation and congenital malformations in the fetus.

Toxicity: Overdoses of manganese usually result from inhalation of manganese dust in a work situation. In children, chronic toxicity has been found to cause learning disabilities.

Interactions: Manganese increases copper excretion from the body. Supplemental iron can interfere with manganese absorption. Food processing destroys manganese content.

Sources: Manganese is plentiful in whole grains and cereals, nuts, seeds and vegetables.

MOLYBDENUM

RDA: No RDA is given for molybdenum by the National Research Council, but a daily dietary intake of 75 to 250 µg/day for adults is suggested as safe and adequate. Additional molybdenum is not needed during pregnancy.

Supplementation: The human requirement for molybdenum is so low that it is easily furnished by most diets.

During Pregnancy: Molybdenum is part of several enzymes and is also found in tooth enamel. However, it plays no role specifically in pregnancy.

Deficiency: Deficiencies have been linked to male infertility and can produce symptoms of neurological damage if prolonged. However, deficiencies are extremely uncommon in the United States and have only been artificially produced in animals.

Toxicity: It takes about 500 µg/day to result in a loss of copper through the urine. More than 1,000 µg/day can induce a gout-like condition.

Interactions: Too much molybdenum interferes with copper metabolism. Processing food decreases its molybdenum content.

Sources: The amount of molybdenum available in the diet depends upon the richness of the soil in which the foods were grown, but it is most likely to be found in legumes, breads and cereals, whole grains, green leafy vegetables, nuts and pineapples.

PARA-AMINOBENZOIC ACID (PABA)

RDA: The RDA for para-aminobenzoic acid has not yet established by the National Research Council.

Supplementation: Due to the toxicity of PABA, supplements should be used with caution, especially if the dosage nears 30 mg.

During Pregnancy: PABA is a part of the B vitamin complex which is stored in all body tissues. PABA has used to treat sunburn, parasitic diseases such as Rocky Mountain spotted fever, and schizophrenia. It is an important component in skin health.

Deficiency: A deficiency (likely to happen only in the presence of sulfa drugs) can result in a variety of symptoms such as fatigue, irritability, depression, nervousness, headache, constipation and other digestive disorders.

Toxicity: High doses of PABA (over 30 mg) can be toxic to the liver, heart and kidneys.

Interactions: A PABA deficiency may result from the use of sulfa drugs, because sulfas resemble PABA in structure and use this similarity to kill intestinal bacteria by substituting for the PABA they need.

Sources: PABA is found in wheat germ, yogurt, molasses and green leafy vegetables.

PHOSPHORUS

RDA: The RDA for phosphorus is 1,200 mg/day; which is established to equal the calcium requirement.

Supplementation: Because almost all foods contain phosphorus, it is rarely included in nutritional supplements, either for pregnancy or generally. About 70 percent of phosphorus from food is absorbed directly from the small intestine into the bloodstream.

During Pregnancy: Phosphorus is an essential part of healthy bones. It is necessary for proper kidney functioning and is involved in the transference of nerve impulses. Phosphorus works with calcium during pregnancy to promote normal cell division and reproduction, bone growth and tooth formation, and to pass along hereditary traits from parents to child. The mother is absorbing and storing greater amounts by the fourth month, but phosphorus is transferred to the fetus primarily during the last three months of pregnancy. Premature babies often need additional phosphorus due to the rate of bone growth required.

Deficiency: Signs of severe phosphorus deficiency include lack of appetite, weight loss or weight gain, irregular breathing, physical fatigue and nervous disorders. A chronic deficiency in a fetus may result in stunted growth, poor teeth and other bone disorders. A phosphorus deficiency can result in a calcium deficit, since the two must be balanced. Processed foods are quite high in phosphorus, without any calcium to balance it. Aluminum hydroxide in antacids can cause a deficiency by binding the phosphorus and making it unavailable.

Toxicity: Extra phosphorus is usually carried out of the body in urine. If the phosphorus level is too high to be controlled by urinary excretion, it will bind calcium in the gastrointestinal tract, thus limiting calcium absorption. The higher the ratio between phosphorus and calcium, the more calcium is excreted in the urine. The presence of vitamin D may help to regulate this process.

Interactions: Phosphorus absorption depends on the presence of vitamin D and calcium. Too much iron, aluminum or magnesium can interfere with phosphorus absorption. White sugar upsets the phosphorus-calcium balance.

Sources: All foods contain phosphorus. Meat, including chicken and fish, contains 15 to 20 times more phosphorus than calcium. This is twice the ratio found in grains, nuts and legumes. Milk, green leafy vegetables and "natural cheeses" contain more calcium than phosphorus. A vegetarian diet requires less calcium and less phosphorus. Less phosphorus is consumed as meats are omitted from the diet. This decreases the calcium need as well, which is why a healthy vegetarian diet does not need milk.

POTASSIUM

RDA: No RDA for potassium has been established, even though a minimum requirement of 3,500 mg per day is recommended by the National Research Council in the latest edition of the RDA. Sufficient potassium is available in the diet naturally, so no call for additional amounts is necessary during pregnancy.

Supplementation: No potassium supplementation is recommended for pregnancy. It is more important to eat plenty of fresh fruits and vegetables. For example, most people who eat a banana a day keep potassium deficiencies away.

During Pregnancy: Potassium is essential to normal growth of the muscle and bone cells, proper activity of the nerve impulses, and good health of the skin. In pregnancy, it helps determine fluid levels in the body, but no studies on the role of potassium in fetal development have been done since fetal deficiencies and toxicities of this mineral are unlikely.

Deficiency: Because a balance must be maintained between potassium and sodium in the body, a potassium deficiency is easily caused by excessive intake of sodium. For example, table salt is very high in sodium but very low in potassium, and a common culprit when potassium levels are low. A potassium deficiency during pregnancy can also result from ongoing morning-sickness vomiting. Alcohol and caffeine increase potassium loss, mostly because they increase urination, which is the primary way the body excretes potassium.

Deficient potassium levels can result in nervous disorders, insomnia, constipation and impaired glucose metabolism, all of which can make pregnancy unpleasant. Prolonged potassium deficiencies will result in impairment of neuromuscular functioning. Potassium is used to treat high blood pressure, so it's important to have it available in the diet in sufficient quantities during pregnancy, particularly if edema (swelling of ankles) occurs.

Toxicity: An excess of potassium can result in cardiac arrest, although urination must be blocked and clinical doses of potassium taken (e.g., high supplemental levels) to be toxic. More than 6,000 mg per day is considered to be a high intake.

Interactions: The balance between sodium and potassium levels in the body is crucial to proper regulation of water balance within the body on the cellular level. Therefore high intake of sodium requires increased intake of potassium. During pregnancy, when fluid levels increase dramatically in the mother's body, this balance is essential.

Sources: All vegetables, particularly green leafy vegetables, whole grains and potatoes (especially potato skin) are good sources of potassium. Potassium is available to some extent in all fresh fruits as well. Vegetarians, who are more likely to eat large amounts of fresh vegetables and fruits, are unlikely to have any potassium deficiencies.

PROTEIN

RDA: Pregnant women are advised to have 60 gr/day, an increase of 10 to 15 gr/day over recommendations prior to pregnancy. The most recent publication of the RDA (1989) by the National Research Council updates protein requirements from its 1980 recommendations in two ways. One is the method by which protein needs are calculated. Before pregnancy, the protein allowance for an adult woman was set at 0.8 gr/kg of body weight per day, or 0.36 gr/lb. The other change relates to the recommended increase in protein intake during pregnancy. The previous RDA (1980) suggested an additional 30 grams of protein be added daily, but now this has been reduced to only 10 grams of extra protein daily during pregnancy.

Supplementation: Increasing dietary protein is sometimes recommended if early signs of toxemia are present, because of a possible role of protein deficiency in pregnancy-induced hypertension. But adding dietary protein is safer than using protein concentrates. Research has found an association linking protein supplementation with an increase in miscarriages and prematurely born infants.

During Pregnancy: Protein is essential to the growth and development of all body tissues, muscles, blood, skin, hair, nails and internal organs, including the heart and the brain. It is important in blood clotting and necessary for the formation of milk during lactation. Additional protein is required during pregnancy by both the mother and the baby. The placenta usually does not transfer protein directly to the fetus. Instead, the fetus synthesizes its own proteins from available amino acids.

The efficiency of maternal protein synthesis increases to almost 70 percent during pregnancy to support expansion of the blood supply, uterus and breasts. Only infants process protein as effectively. In addition to more efficient synthesis, pregnant women store protein in their skeletal muscle. With the naturally increased appetite of pregnancy, the requirement of 10 additional grams of protein a day will be easily satisfied.

Deficiency: Pregnant women are more likely to have caloric deficiencies than protein deficits. While protein deficiency can lead to abnormalities of growth and tissue development, the diet will almost always show a lack of sufficient calories as well. Research has shown that increasing complex carbohydrate intake (e.g., whole grains and cereals) was just as effective in raising birth weight as providing additional protein alone. Protein deficiency has been linked to pregnancy-induced hypertension, but the strength of the link is hotly debated.

Toxicity: The amount of carbohydrates in plant protein foods provides a natural limitation to quantity of protein ingested (you'll feel full before overdoing protein intake when you eat protein from plant foods). Too much protein by itself can be as harmful as too little. Supplements with more than 20 percent of the calories from protein have been associated with retarded fetal growth, whereas supplements with less than 20 percent of calories from protein increase birth weight.

Interactions: To a surprising extent, people are able to adapt well to a lower protein diet, provided carbohydrate intake is sufficient. Meat carries health risks such as higher cholesterol and atherosclerosis. Protein needs are affected by energy use, through exercise and through the pregnancy process itself.

Sources: Protein is found in legumes, nuts, seeds and root vegetables. It is also quite plentiful in whole grain breads, cereals and pastas and, to a lesser extent, in other vegetables. Sprouting grains and beans will increase protein digestibility, levels of folic acid, ascorbic acid and the bioavailability of iron in the seeds. The following protein sources are probably found in your diet:

2 tbs peanut butter	8.0 grams
¼ cup peanuts	9.5 grams
½ cup wheat germ	16.5 grams
½ cup wild rice	11.3 grams
½ cup lentils	8.5 grams
½ cup black beans	22.0 grams
½ cup pinto beans	21.5 grams
1 cup soy milk	10.0 grams
4 oz tofu	20.0 grams
4 oz whole wheat pasta	20.0 grams

SELENIUM

RDA: The RDA for selenium is 65 µg/day, up 10 µg/day from 55 µg/day for non-pregnant adult women. The RDA increases to 75 µg during lactation.

Supplementation: No need is indicated for laboratory tests to assess selenium status during pregnancy or to advise pregnant women to take supplemental selenium, according to the final report to the federal government by the Subcommittee on Dietary Intake and Nutrient Supplements during Pregnancy.

During Pregnancy: Selenium is an essential mineral, but this was only determined in 1979. Selenium preserves tissue elasticity, protects against high blood pressure and strokes, slows down the aging process, prevents cataracts and relieves arthritis. Selenium is essential for reproduction and male sperm cells contain high amounts of it. The liver and kidneys contain four to five times as much selenium as muscles and other tissues. Although individual eating habits differ considerably, the body can adjust its own selenium levels as necessary within a wide range of dietary patterns. Minor excesses of selenium in the diet are excreted in the urine.

Deficiency: Research shows that a clinically induced selenium deficiency can result in infertility, impotency and premature aging. A selenium deficiency occurs only when vitamin E is also missing from the diet. Increasing vitamin E intake counteracts the symptoms of a selenium deficiency. Deficiencies are unlikely because homeostatic control of selenium is very strong.

Toxicity: Selenium can potentially exert toxic effects on a fetus. Symptoms of supplement overdoses include nausea, abdominal pain, diarrhea, nail and hair changes, fatigue and irritability. There are several different selenium compounds, some more toxic than others. Sodium selenite is more toxic than organic selenium, selenium yeast is a third as toxic as sodium selenite, and dimethyl selenium is non-toxic.

Interactions: Selenium works closely with vitamin E in metabolic actions and in the promotion of normal body growth and fertility. A deficiency of one can be prevented or cured by supplementation of the other. Sulfur from fertilizers and acid rain can inhibit plant absorption of the mineral from the soil. Selenium in foods is easily reduced up to 50 percent by heat, processing and cooking. Selenium is combined with protein to treat kwashiorkor.

Sources: Grains and seeds have significant amounts of selenium, although the selenium in almost all plant foods depends upon the soil in which the plants are grown. Brewer's yeast and wheat germ are rich in selenium.

SODIUM

RDA: Because people usually get far more sodium than they need, no RDA has been established for it, but no less than 2 to 3 grams of sodium should be available daily.

Supplementation: Sodium is so easily available that it is not included in pregnancy or other nutritional supplements.

During Pregnancy: Sodium is an essential mineral found primarily in bodily fluids. It regulates water balance and distribution of bodily fluids, keeps blood minerals soluble, and facilitates the digestive process. Because fluids increase in the mother during pregnancy, the amount of sodium must also increase to keep her system balanced. Doctors used to recommend restriction of salt at any sign of edema, but salt restriction during pregnancy has proven to do more harm than good. Moderate edema is normal during pregnancy and should not be combated with diuretics and low-sodium diets. Sodium has been used to treat diarrhea, adrenal exhaustion, leg cramps, tooth and gum disorders, and dehydration.

Deficiency: It is very rare to find someone with a sodium deficiency since it's found in almost all foods. However, a sodium deficiency can cause intestinal gas, weight loss and vomiting. Carbohydrate conversion into fat is impaired when sodium is absent. Macrobiotic vegetarians who strictly restrict sodium intake have had problems with digestion, since sodium is so essential to the digestive process. Kelp and other sea vegetables have a reasonably high sodium content naturally, as does soy sauce. These should be a part of any normal diet that otherwise limits sodium intake.

Toxicity: Sodium content is highest in processed foods and, of course, table salt. Usually 90 to 95 percent of sodium that is ingested is excreted in the urine. Too much sodium may cause potassium loss and abnormal fluid retention. More than 14 grams a day of sodium chloride is considered excessive.

Sources: Sodium is found naturally in sea vegetables, particularly kelp. It is available in small (safe) quantities in almost every food.

VITAMIN A

RDA: The RDA for adult females is 800 µg/day. No additional amount of vitamin A is needed during pregnancy, but the RDA is increased by 500 µg/day during lactation. Vitamin A levels are measured both in retinol equivalents (RE) and international units (IU). Because the RE measurement takes into consideration the absorption rate of the kind of vitamin A ingested and is therefore more accurate, it is the standard unit now in use.

Supplementation: Since the RDA for vitamin A does not increase during pregnancy, no supplement is necessary if you get sufficient amounts in your diet already. However, vitamin A is frequently included in pregnancy supplements anyway because most diets in the United States are low in vitamin A-rich foods (fruits and vegetables.) But overdoses of vitamin A are also one of the most common problems of self-supplementation during pregnancy. Vitamin A supplements for pregnant women should not exceed 10,000 µg/day.

During Pregnancy: Vitamin A is mostly absorbed in the upper intestinal tract approximately four to six hours after ingestion. It is important for cell differentiation and fetal growth—deficiencies are associated with smaller babies and pre-term births. Vitamin A is fat-soluble and can be stored in fatty tissues, lungs, kidneys and the retina. Vitamin A crosses the placenta and is stored in fetal liver tissue. Vitamin A will continue to build up in the fetus as long as maternal levels are high, so it is important not to exceed the RDA (excess vitamin A is not good for the fetus or the mother.)

Deficiency: Vitamin A deficiency can be devastating to fetal development but is rarely observed during pregnancy. A possible explanation for this may be that a woman with a vitamin A deficiency may be more likely to miscarry in the earliest stages—possibly even before the woman knows she is pregnant. Infertile women should be sure that their vitamin A intake level is adequate. Males may have trouble with semen potency if their diets are deficient in vitamin A. Severe vitamin A deficiencies during pregnancy can result in babies who are born with microcephaly, or eye and vision impairments.

Toxicity: Vitamin A is a powerful substance and should not be taken in excess as a way of assuring adequacy—too much vitamin A is just as harmful to fetal development as too little. Excesses can cause spontaneous abortions, or head, heart and nervous system malformations. The carotene form of vitamin A (found in fruits and vegetables) usually is not harmful in large amounts since it is less efficiently absorbed. For example, a large carrot has about 11,000 IU of carotene, and is perfectly safe to eat. A comparable amount in a supplement form goes beyond the recommended safety limit because the concentrated form will affect the body in one dose, rather than through the normal digestive cycle with food fibers as a buffer.

Interactions: Excessive iron interferes with the absorption of vitamin A. Zinc must be present for the liver to extract vitamin A from storage tissues. A diet low in fat will cause vitamin A to be excreted more quickly in the feces.

Sources: Vitamin A is found in all fruits and vegetables. If you eat six or more servings of fruits and vegetables a day, your vitamin A intake will be sufficient.

VITAMIN B₁/THIAMINE

RDA: During pregnancy, the RDA is 1.5 mg/day, up from the 1.1 mg recommended prior to conception.

Supplementation: Thiamine is usually included in pregnancy supplements since the need for this nutrient is known to increase during gestation.

During Pregnancy: Thiamine is one of the B complex vitamins. It improves food assimilation and digestion, particularly of starches, sugars and alcohol. If carbohydrate intake increases, the amount of thiamine absorbed also increases. Thiamine is necessary for consistent growth in children and good muscle tone in stomach, intestines and heart. Thiamine is not stored in the body and must be part of a daily diet. Requirements for this nutrient increase during pregnancy because of the increased caloric intake of the first half and the needs of the fetus in the last half.

Deficiency: A deficiency of thiamine makes it harder to digest carbohydrates. Signs of deficiency include easy fatigue and mood swings. A thiamine deficiency can occur in the mother without visible signs, but it will result in the baby being born with reduced stores of the nutrient and less ability to fight off beriberi. (Should this occur, intravenous injections of thiamine will improve the baby's condition rapidly.)

Thiamine deficiencies have been found in a proportion of pregnant women everywhere, both in well-nourished communities and in areas where the diet is generally considered deficient. A deficiency is most common in societies that consume a high proportion of white rice, because the process of making white rice refines out the thiamine (as well as other essential nutrients). As a rule, rice should be unrefined for fullest nutrient value, although enriched white rices are available.

Toxicity: There are no known toxic effects of excess thiamine, although large amounts alone may cause other B vitamin imbalances.

Interactions: Thiamine is vulnerable to heat, air and water in cooking. Eating sugar, smoking and drinking alcohol can cause a thiamine depletion.

Sources: Thiamine is found in unrefined cereal grains, brewer's yeast, and some seeds and nuts.

VITAMIN B$_2$/RIBOFLAVIN

RDA: The RDA for B$_2$ is 1.6 mg daily, up from 1.3 mg recommended before conception. Lactation raises the recommendation higher, to 1.8 mg/day during the first six months of nursing.

Supplementation: Since the need for B$_2$ increases slightly during pregnancy, it is often included in supplements.

During Pregnancy: Vitamin B$_2$, also known as riboflavin, is a water-soluble vitamin occurring naturally in foods that contain other B vitamins. It works with digestive enzymes to break down carbohydrates, fats and proteins, as well as helping cells use oxygen. It is important for healthy vision, skin, hair and nails. B$_2$ is not stored in the body and requirements are influenced by the caloric intake of the individual. It is easily absorbed through the wall of the small intestine, and then carried in the blood to various tissues throughout the body. Excess riboflavin is excreted in the urine.

Vitamin B$_2$ is actively transported by the placenta to the fetus. It is one of the few nutrients that appears to increase naturally when blood volume expands during pregnancy. The amount of riboflavin excreted in the urine decreases during the third trimester, suggesting that more riboflavin is used by the fetus during that time.

Deficiency: Prolonged use of oral contraceptives (over one year) causes a riboflavin deficiency. Women in the third trimester of pregnancy who get too little B$_2$ often suffer from visual disturbances, burning sensations in the eyes, excessive watering of the eyes, failing vision and the like. These conditions are helped by supplements.

A vitamin B$_2$ deficiency may also be connected to a higher incidence of vomiting and premature deliveries. Problems with lactation and nursing are more common if a B$_2$ deficiency is present in the mother after giving birth.

Toxicity: There is no known toxic level of riboflavin, but excesses (out of proportion to other B vitamin intake) may result in loss of other B vitamins in urine.

Interactions: Riboflavin is stable in the presence of heat, oxidation and acid, but disintegrates in alkali or light, particularly ultraviolet light.

Sources: Riboflavin is found naturally in brewer's yeast but is scarce elsewhere in plant foods. "Enriched" grains, breads and cereals usually contain B$_2$.

VITAMIN B$_3$/NIACIN

RDA: The RDA for niacin is 17 mg/day during pregnancy, up from 13 mg/day for non-pregnant women. It increases to 20 mg/day during the first months of nursing.

Supplementation: An increase in niacin is recommended during pregnancy to meet higher energy needs, so this nutrient is often included in pregnancy supplements. Always take a supplement containing B_3 on a full stomach since niacin is involved in the release of stomach acid.

During Pregnancy: There are three synthetic forms of niacin: niacinamide, nicotinic acid and nicotinamide. Vitamin B_3 is a water-soluble vitamin that is absorbed in the intestine and stored in the liver. Necessary for the formation and maintenance of healthy skin, tongue and digestive system tissues, it is also used in the synthesis of sex hormones, for improving circulation and for proper activity of the nervous system. Supplemental B_3 can be used to treat health problems such as migraines, diarrhea, atherosclerosis and high blood pressure.

Few studies have been done regarding changes in niacin levels during pregnancy, partly because of the difficulty in accurately testing for this vitamin. Levels of niacin in urinary excretion increase through pregnancy, to almost twice the normal rate. This is probably because, during pregnancy, a good deal of tryptophan is converted by the body into niacin, resulting in extra niacin. This decreases the need for niacin from dietary sources.

Deficiency: A B_3 deficiency can have many effects, including muscular weakness, general fatigue, loss of appetite, indigestion and skin problems. Too little niacin can cause fetal malformations and miscarriages, so a minimum level in the diet is important. However, since the body creates excess niacin from tryptophan during pregnancy, it is unlikely that niacin deficiencies will be encountered.

Toxicity: Excesses of B_3 in the form of niacinamide can cause depression and liver damage. Other forms show no toxic effects, but over 100 mg/day may cause some side effects due to a dilation of the blood vessels. Excess is usually controlled through urinary excretion.

Interactions: Niacin is more stable than thiamine or riboflavin and remarkably resistant to heat, light, air, acids and alkalis. Excessive consumption of sugar, starches or antibiotics will deplete the body's stores.

Sources: Brewer's yeast, peanuts and wheat germ are high in niacin. Tryptophan is a component of protein and even a small amount of it can be converted into sufficient niacin in the body.

VITAMIN B$_5$/PANTOTHENIC ACID

RDA: While listing no RDA for vitamin B$_5$, the National Research Council does give an "estimated safe and adequate daily allowance" of 4 to 7 mg. This is not increased for pregnancy or lactation.

Supplementation: Because there is no RDA for vitamin B$_5$ and because the estimated safe allowance does not increase for pregnancy, supplementation is not considered necessary. However, because it is part of the B vitamin complex, it is sometimes included in pregnancy and B vitamin supplements.

During Pregnancy: Pantothenic acid is a B complex vitamin, important in facilitating the release of energy from carbohydrates. It is water-soluble, and may be synthesized by intestinal bacteria flora. Pantothenic acid is essential for proper functioning of the gastrointestinal tract: intestinal gas and abdominal distension can be relieved by supplements of this nutrient. The brain has one of the highest concentrations of B_5 of all systems in the body. Vitamin B_5 may be beneficial for cystitis, diarrhea, insomnia, mental illness, adrenal exhaustion and flatulence.

Little is known about the specific role of pantothenic acid in pregnancy, although changes in the digestive system during this time must involve this nutrient in some way. If pregnant women need greater amounts of pantothenate than non-pregnant women, extra amounts are easily obtained from food.

Deficiency: A B_5 deficiency can spur a broad spectrum of biochemical defects including infertility and spontaneous abortions, but deficiencies do not occur except in cases of malnutrition. Stress may decrease B_5 and a deficiency may cause exhaustion of the adrenal gland, resulting in physical and mental depression.

Toxicity: B_5 is relatively non-toxic, but large amounts (10 to 20 grams/day) may produce occasional diarrhea and water retention.

Interactions: Fifty percent of B_5 content in grains is lost through the milling process. Vitamin B_5 is easily destroyed by acid (vinegar) or alkali (baking soda). Stress, illness and antibiotic medicines increase the need for pantothenic acid.

Sources: Vitamin B_5 is widely available in foods, especially whole grain cereals and legumes.

VITAMIN B_6/PYRIDOXINE

RDA: The RDA for vitamin B_6 is 2.2 mg/day during pregnancy, up from 1.6 mg recommended for women before pregnancy. This amount decreases very slightly, to 2.1 mg/day during lactation.

Supplementation: Vitamin B_6 is often included in dietary supplements since the need for it increases during pregnancy. A supplement is sometimes given to reduce severe nausea: Adele Davis recommended 10 mg of vitamin B_6 daily for a month or two before pregnancy to avoid nausea, or 250 mg daily during pregnancy if nausea had already started. Supplementation may also be helpful to women with previous births of cleft-palate children.

During Pregnancy: Vitamin B_6 is a water-soluble vitamin that helps to maintain the balance of sodium and potassium in the body. B_6 is composed of three compounds that may internally adjust themselves for maximum efficiency of use by the maternal body. B_6 is excreted from the body within eight hours after ingestion. During pregnancy, the mother's body retains more B_6, suggesting that her need for the vitamin has risen.

Deficiency: When they are expecting, most women will show a natural deficiency of vitamin B_6, which even a supplement of 10 mg/day in early pregnancy will not prevent. In some women, the first weeks of pregnancy are marked by nausea and the mother loses her appetite and/or her ability to keep food down. Many of these early morning-sickness signs are also symptoms of a vitamin B_6 deficiency and some evidence shows that a B_6 supplement will ease them. If the deficiency gets worse in late pregnancy, the risk of stillbirths and post-delivery infant mortality increases.

Toxicity: If B_6 is ingested out of proportion to other B vitamins, this will cause deficiencies of other B vitamins. Taken in large dosages by itself over a period of years, it can cause sensory and neuropathological damage. However, toxicity from foods high in B_6 is rare, because other B vitamins are usually present as well and excesses of B_6 are usually excreted daily in the urine.

Interactions: Radiation, oral contraceptives and aging increase the need for B_6. Too much B_6 without sufficient zinc can lead to numbness and tingling of extremities.

Sources: Vitamin B_6 is found in nutritional yeast, blackstrap molasses, wheat germ, cantaloupe, bananas and avocados.

VITAMIN B_{12}/CYANOCOBALAMIN

RDA: The RDA for vitamin B_{12} increases .2 µg/day during pregnancy, to a total of 2.2 µg/day. During lactation, the RDA increases again to 2.6 µg/day. The daily requirement for B_{12} was lowered by one third in the most recent (10th) edition of the RDA and still is twice the safe level established by the FAO (Food and Agriculture Organization, in conjunction with the World Health Organization) in 1988. The change was based on the lack of evidence to support the need for maintaining a large reservoir of the vitamin in the body.

Supplementation: A vitamin B_{12} supplement or foods fortified with B_{12} are recommended for all vegan diets, since B_{12} is essential to the health of the nervous system. During pregnancy, vitamin B_{12} is a vital nutrient to include in a supplement if you have any doubt that your diet provides sufficient amounts.

During Pregnancy: Vitamin B_{12} is a water-soluble vitamin that cannot be made synthetically; it is manufactured by bacteria, fungi or algae. Vitamin B_{12} is necessary for normal cell division and protein synthesis during pregnancy. There is a natural decline in B_{12} serum levels that is not prevented by supplemental doses of B_{12}. At the same time, intestinal capacity to absorb B_{12} is increased during pregnancy, and the placenta concentrates the vitamin so that babies at birth have double their mothers' level of vitamin B$_{12}$.

Excess vitamin B$_{12}$ is stored by the human body for up to 30 years. Vitamin B$_{12}$ is a nutrient found in animal foods, but not directly in plant foods unless it's deliberately added. If you have eaten any animal foods (meat, eggs, dairy) within the last five years, you probably have enough already available and do not need a supplement. However, if your body is deficient due to previous stress or other drains on B$_{12}$, you may not have stored enough B$_{12}$ for the intestines to use efficiently.

Deficiency: Deficiencies may take years to become evident since the body stores this vitamin for so long and requires very little. Although a mother may not show a vitamin B$_{12}$ deficiency, her baby may be born with one. An innate deficiency of this vitamin will put the newborn more at risk for illness. Taking supplemental B$_{12}$ during pregnancy will assure your baby of sufficient bodily stores at birth.

B$_{12}$ intake has been a concern of vegetarians and researchers alike, since it is the one nutrient that is available almost solely in animal products. Fermented soy products were reputed to have B$_{12}$, but modern processing methods destroy the bacteria that produce the nutrient. Recent research also indicates that seaweeds do not have available B$_{12}$, as had been previously thought.

Toxicity: No cases of vitamin B$_{12}$ overdoses or toxicity have been reported.

Interactions: High folic acid may mask a vitamin B$_{12}$ deficiency. Absorption is decreased by 5 to 10 percent when large amounts are taken. Absorption rate increases naturally during pregnancy. Laxatives and iron and calcium deficiencies will reduce available vitamin B$_{12}$ stores in the body.

Sources: A vitamin B_{12} supplement, some fermented soy products (which contain the mold necessary for B_{12} to grow), and foods fortified with B_{12} (soy milks, soy yogurts, brewer's yeast) will provide this vitamin.

VITAMIN B_{15}/PANGAMIC ACID

RDA: Due to a lack of evidence that B_{15} (also known as pangamic acid) is an essential nutrient, no RDA has been established for it by the National Research Council.

Supplementation: Since no RDA is set for this nutrient, supplementation is considered unnecessary.

During Pregnancy: Pangamic acid, also known as vitamin B_{15}, is a water-soluble nutrient originally isolated in apricot kernels. It is thought to be active in cell respiration and protein metabolism. Pangamic acid has been suggested in the treatment of such problems as circulatory disturbances, high cholesterol and emphysema. It may help in the prevention of cancer, but a definite link has not been established. There are no known effects of this nutrient on pregnancy.

Deficiency: No undesirable effects have resulted from a deficiency of this nutrient, although some studies suggest a connection between a deficiency and heart disease and nervous system disorders.

Toxicity: Toxicity of vitamin B_{15} is reached at 100,000 times the therapeutic dosage of 100 mg/day. Excesses are excreted through sweat, the kidneys and the bowels.

Interactions: Little is known about the process of B_{15} absorption or about its interactions with other nutrients and foods.

Sources: Vitamin B$_{15}$ is found in brewer's yeast, whole grains and cereals, sesame seeds and pumpkin seeds.

VITAMIN C/ASCORBIC ACID

RDA: The RDA for vitamin C is set at 70 mg/day, an increase of 10 mg/day during pregnancy. During lactation the RDA increases to 95 mg/day.

Supplementation: Vitamin C is usually included in a pregnancy or other supplement because it facilitates absorption of the A, E and the B complex vitamins.

During Pregnancy: Vitamin C is a water-soluble nutrient and an antioxidant whose primary function is to maintain collagen, a protein used to form connective tissue. Vitamin C aids in forming red blood cells, preventing hemorrhaging and reducing allergic responses. It fights infections and viruses and stimulates the immune system. Vitamin C converts folic acid to an active form, protects A, E and B vitamins from oxidation. Vitamin C reaches its maximum level in the blood two to three hours after ingestion. Excess vitamin C carried to the bladder may prevent bladder cancer. Vitamin C can be synthesized by many mammals, but not by humans.

The plasma concentration of vitamin C normally drops by 25 to 40 percent as a woman approaches term. This may be caused by plasma volume expansion and the resulting dilution. Fetal and infant plasma levels are 50 percent higher than maternal stores, so it likely that fetal stores are adequate for proper development despite this dilution.

Deficiency: Symptoms of deficiency include impaired digestion, poor lactation, bleeding gums, weakened teeth, tendency to bruising, swollen and painful joints, nosebleeds and lowered resistance to infection. Vitamin C deficiency has been associated with an increased frequency of premature labor. Healthy vegetarian diets are high in vitamin C-rich fruits and vegetables, so this is less likely to be a problem encountered by vegetarian mothers.

Toxicity: Too much vitamin C (over 600 mg/day) may cause a spontaneous abortion or miscarriage in the earliest stages of pregnancy. Excessive vitamin C during pregnancy has been linked with the development of scurvy after birth in the infant.

Interactions: Lower levels of vitamin C were found in women taking oral contraceptives. While vitamin C is fairly stable in acid solutions (such as fruit juice), typically it is the least stable of all vitamins. Ascorbic acid is sensitive to oxygen, light, heat and air. Vitamin C-rich foods should not be left at room temperature after they have been cut and prepared for eating. Vitamin C is used up quickly during times of emotional stress, since large concentrations are needed by the adrenal glands. Alcohol and smoking destroy it. The presence of vitamin C greatly increases intestinal absorption of iron.

Sources: Vitamin C is found in fruits, particularly citrus fruits and mangoes, and in green vegetables such as broccoli, kale and green peppers.

VITAMIN D/CALCIFEROL

RDA: The RDA for vitamin D increases 5 µg/day (200 IU) to 10 µg/day (400 IU) for pregnant women, with no additional increase for lactation.

Supplementation: A 10 µg/day supplement of vitamin D is recommended by the National Research Council for pregnant vegans and a 5 µg/day supplement for those who drink only a little milk. Two forms of vegetarian vitamin D supplements can be purchased. Vitamin D_2, also called calciferol or ergocalciferol or activated ergosterol, is prepared by ultraviolet irradiation of ergosterol derived from yeast. This form of vitamin D could be called vegan. Vitamin D_3 is prepared by irradiation of 7-dehydrocholesterol derived from lanolin from sheep's or lamb's wool and so is a supplemental form many vegetarians would want to avoid.

During Pregnancy: Vitamin D is a fat-soluble vitamin which can be stored by the body. It works with calcium and phosphorus in bone and tooth formation, and increases its capacity to make both calcium and phosphorus more available during pregnancy. Fetal need for vitamin D has not been determined. But calcium is deposited in the fetus, so an assumption can be made that additional vitamin D may also be necessary for proper fetal development.

Deficiency: If the mother's diet is deficient in vitamin D, the rate of calcium absorption will be lowered, also lowering the amount of calcium available to both mother and child. A fetus is likely to develop clinical signs of the deficiency (poor bone and tooth formation, rickets in the womb) before the mother shows any obvious deficiencies. A deficiency in the mother during the last trimester can affect the development of tooth enamel, producing weaker teeth in the baby. In winter, the ultraviolet light reaching the earth's surface has been found to be insufficient for vitamin D synthesis in the skin in such places as Britain, Canada (Edmonton) and even Massachusetts.

Toxicity: Too much vitamin D (more than five times the RDA) can be toxic. If you are out in the sun a lot during your pregnancy or drink more than three glasses of vitamin D-enriched milk a day, a vitamin D supplement may be detrimental rather than helpful. Recently, an article in the *New England Journal of Medicine* reported that 13 brands of vitamin D-fortified milk in the northeast United States were found to have vitamin D levels that were well below or appreciably above the suggested dosage. Eight patients were hospitalized when one dairy added vitamin D in toxic amounts. High vitamin D levels during pregnancy have been associated with mental and physical retardation in infants.

Interactions: Vitamin D is closely involved with the metabolism of calcium, phosphorus and magnesium, and all these nutrients must be present in adequate amounts for any one of them to work efficiently. A vitamin D deficiency lowers the rate of calcium absorption for both mother and child.

Sources: Sunlight (at least half an hour a day on arms, legs and face) can provide sufficient vitamin D. Vitamin D-fortified foods are the only non-animal sources of this vitamin.

VITAMIN E/TOCOPHEROL

RDA: The RDA for vitamin E is 10 IU daily, up from a preconception RDA of 8 IU/day. This figure goes up to 12 IU/day during the first six months of nursing.

Supplementation: According to the National Research Council, vitamin E supplements are not necessary for most pregnant women. However, premature infants are routinely given supplemental E.

During Pregnancy: Vitamin E is a fat-soluble vitamin stored in bile salts and fat, and composed of several tocopherols: alpha, beta, gamma, delta, epsilon, zeta and eta, named for the first seven letters of the Greek alphabet. Vitamin E is an antioxidant, protecting the body from the formation of molecules involved in cancer, blood clots and DNA damage from environmental poisons. Vitamin E helps skin tissue heal without scarring and has been shown to be successful in treating varicose veins. During pregnancy, vitamin E may help to increase fertility in both men and women, and to maintain the pregnancy, preventing miscarriages and spontaneous abortions.

Deficiency: A problem with vitamin E absorption must persist for 5 to 10 years before neurological damage starts to appear. Deficiencies of vitamin E are unlikely in most diets, but serious deficiencies can lead to muscular and digestive problems, and decrease the survival of red blood cells. Severe deficiencies in men may lead to degeneration of tissues in the testes which supplementation cannot reverse. Women who are severely deficient in vitamin E are extremely likely to miscarry or have their children prematurely.

Toxicity: Individuals who take large amounts of vitamin E without being accustomed to it may find that their blood pressure rises, so anyone with a tendency to high blood pressure should not take high dosages. But in general, vitamin E is considered safe over a wide range of intakes. No evidence of toxicity was observed in a study of adults given vitamin E supplements of 800 mg/day.

Interactions: Inorganic iron, chlorine in drinking water, ferric chloride and rancid oils destroy vitamin E in the body. Inorganic iron supplements should be taken 8 to 12 hours after a vitamin E supplement. Food processing may destroy vitamin E. Selenium is metabolically involved with vitamin E to the extent that a deficiency of one can be prevented or cured with supplementation of the other.

Sources: Cold-pressed vegetable oils, all whole raw seeds and nuts, soybeans and wheat germ are good natural sources of vitamin E.

VITAMIN K

RDA: The RDA for vitamin K is 60 μg daily for women ages 17 to 24 and 65 μg for women over 24. The RDA for pregnancy and lactation has been set at 60 μg/day. Until the latest edition of the RDAs was published in 1989, no requirement at all had been established for vitamin K.

Supplementation: Since most people get sufficient vitamin K in their diet without effort, and since no additional need has been discovered for this vitamin during pregnancy, a supplement is unnecessary.

During Pregnancy: Vitamin K is a fat-soluble vitamin essential in the process of blood coagulation, a process which is very important during delivery and for proper liver functioning as well. Vitamin K injections are sometimes given to women before labor if hemorrhaging has occurred in previous births. Although most adult women tend to get more than adequate vitamin K in their regular diets (300 to 500 μg/day is average), babies are born with relatively low stores of the vitamin. Some forms of vitamin K are synthesized in the intestines, but only a very limited transfer of the vitamin occurs from mother to child through the placenta.

Many pediatric and obstetric professional groups recommend that 0.5 to 1.0 mg. of vitamin K in the form of phytonadione be given to newborns in a single dose after birth, to make up for the low stores with which most babies are born. This is sometimes followed by another such dose after about a month, since milk does not contain substantial vitamin K.

Deficiency: Vitamin K deficiencies may be a factor in miscarriages. Because vitamin K is necessary for the formation of several proteins involved in the regulation of blood clotting, defective coagulation of the blood is the only major sign of vitamin K deficiency. If you are being treated with antibiotics there is a chance of a vitamin K deficiency. Unfortunately, vitamin K deficiency is only determined by the time it takes for blood to clot, and can often be discovered only in an emergency situation.

Toxicity: No toxic reactions have been observed, even when vitamin K was consumed in large amounts over an extended time period. On the other hand, the *Nutrition Almanac* reports that toxic reactions have been observed when pregnant women were injected with large dosages of synthetic vitamin K.

Interactions: Vitamin K absorption depends on sufficient fat in the diet, so a deficiency of fat can increase problems with proper blood clotting. An excess of vitamin E can produce a vitamin K deficiency in which blood clots more slowly, but blood clotting will normalize with supplementation. Unsaturated fats increase vitamin K production by intestinal flora. Antibiotics, radiation, x-rays, aspirin and industrial air pollution all destroy vitamin K.

Sources: The vitamin K content of most foods is not known with precision. Green leafy vegetables provide 50 to 800 µg of vitamin K per 100 grams of vegetable. Safflower oil, blackstrap molasses, soy foods and cauliflower are also known to contain vitamin K.

ZINC

RDA: The RDA for zinc is 15 mg, up from 12 mg/day for adult non-pregnant women. The RDA rises during nursing to 19 mg/day.

Supplementation: Zinc levels decline somewhat during pregnancy, but supplementation will not prevent this decline. Do not over-supplement, as too much zinc can be toxic.

During Pregnancy: Zinc is a trace mineral occurring in large amounts in the human body, more than any other trace mineral except iron. It is stored throughout the body, from the liver to the bones to the skin, toenails and parts of the eyes. Zinc is necessary for nucleic acid and protein metabolism, cell differentiation and replication. It is essential for proper development of the reproductive organs, general growth, and normal functioning of the prostrate gland. It also increases resistance to infection, improves night vision, and reduces body odor.

Zinc status in the body is regulated by means of homeostatic controls. Adults can adapt to a wide range of zinc intakes. Small amounts of zinc are more efficiently absorbed than large amounts. People with poor zinc status absorb zinc more efficiently than people in good health. Therefore, zinc requirements of an individual depend upon her zinc status. Assessing zinc status is difficult, and not a routine part of pregnancy care.

Zinc has been used to help prevent and treat infertility. During pregnancy, zinc may reduce the incidence of pregnancy-related hypertension by affecting prostaglandin metabolism. Additional zinc may be helpful at birth in the healing process of both internal and external wounds.

Deficiency: Maternal zinc deficiency is harmful to development of the growing baby, directly affecting fetal growth and involving complications during labor, such as prolonged labor and bleeding. There may be immediate impairment of cell growth and repair in response to a zinc deficiency. However, studies of zinc deficiency are contradictory so that undetermined factors may be affecting the results. Stretch marks may occur more easily in the presence of a zinc deficiency; brittle nails, easily broken hair, white spots on the fingernails and fatigue are also indicators of a zinc deficiency. A loss of normal taste sensitivity and appetite may result from a zinc deficiency. Nausea associated with pregnancy may be due to combined deficiencies in zinc and vitamin B_6.

Toxicity: Zinc is primarily excreted through the gastrointestinal tract rather than through urine. A daily zinc intake of 50 mg or more will interfere with copper utilization and cause incomplete iron metabolism, while two grams or more a day may cause gastrointestinal irritation and vomiting. In one study, zinc supplementation of 20 times the RDA resulted in the impairment of various immune responses.

Interactions: Foods that contain high levels of phytic acids, such as bran and whole grains may reduce the absorption rate of zinc. Other foods such as white bread, milk and soy products increase the absorption rate, dependent upon soil content and minimal food processing. Alcohol flushes zinc from the liver into the urine and out of the body; chronic alcohol use will cause a zinc deficiency that will impair fertility. Oral contraceptives lower zinc levels in blood plasma. Increased phosphorus, protein or iron in the diet raise zinc requirements.

Sources: Medical professionals are often concerned with zinc status in a vegetarian diet since zinc is more easily available from animal foods than from plant foods. Whole grain products are believed to have a less available form because of the presence of phytic acid. When calcium level is high, phytic acids are more active. When calcium levels are relatively low, more zinc is absorbed from plant foods. A zinc deficiency is rarely a problem in a vegetarian diet unless calcium intake is high (from excess dairy).

Appendix

LEVELS OF NUTRIENTS

(Toxic levels occur most frequently when supplements are used.)

VITAMINS	RDA for Pregnancy	Toxic Level (per day)
Vitamin A	800 μg	10,000 μg (as supplement)
Vitamin B Complex:		
Biotin	100 to 200 μg	not specified
Choline	not set	not specified
Folic Acid	400 μg	not specified
Inositol	not set	not specified
Para-aminobenzoic acid (PABA)	not set	30 mg
B_1/Thiamine	1.5 mg	not specified
B_2/Riboflavin	1.6 mg	not specified
B_3/Niacin	17 mg	100 mg
B_5/Pantothenic Acid	4.7 mg	10 mg
B_6/Pyridoxine	2.2 mg	not specified
B_{12}/Cyanocobalamin	2.2 μg	not specified
B_{15}/Pangamic Acid	not set	100 mg
Vitamin C/Ascorbic Acid	70 mg	600 mg
Vitamin D/Calciferol	10 μg	50 μg
Vitamin E/Tocopherol	10 mg	not specified
Vitamin K	65 μg	not specified

MINERALS		
Calcium	1,200 mg	not specified
Chlorides	not set	not specified
Chromium	50 to 200 μg	not specified

Copper	1.5 to 3 mg	10 mg
Fluorides	1.5 to 4 mg	10 mg
Iodine	175 μg	not specified
Iron	30 mg	variable
Magnesium	300 mg	not specified
Manganese	2 to 5 mg	10 mg
Molybdenum	75 to 250 μg	500 μg
Phosphorus	1,200 mg	varies with calcium intake
Potassium	3,500 mg	6,000 mg
Selenium	65 μg	1 to 2 mg
Sodium	not set	14 g
Zinc	15 mg	50 mg

References:

Dunne, Lavon J., *Nutrition Almanac, 3rd edition,* McGraw-Hill, New York, NY, 1990.

Institute of Medicine, *Nutrition During Pregnancy,* National Academy Press, Washington, DC, 1990.

National Research Council, *Recommended Daily Allowances, 10th edition,* National Academy Press, Washington, DC, 1990.

Glossary of Terms

abortifacient. A drug or other agent that causes abortion.

amniotic fluids. Fluids in the embryonic sac (in the uterus) that surround the growing fetus.

Apgar score. A rating with a maximum score of ten used to measure the vital signs of a newborn in the first minute after birth. A score over seven indicates a healthy baby.

atherosclerosis. Deposits of small fatty nodules on the inner walls of the arteries which hamper normal blood flow.

beriberi. A disease characterized by nerve disorders which is caused by the lack of vitamin B_1 (thiamine) in the diet.

bilirubin. The yellowish-red pigment of human bile normally found in small quantities in blood and urine; high concentrations will show up as discoloration of blood and urine, resulting in jaundice and indicating a breakdown or destruction of the red blood cells.

bio-availablility. The degree to which a nutrient enters the bloodstream and is circulated to various body organs and tissues.

Bradley method. A method of natural childbirth developed by Dr. Robert A. Bradley from the principles of Dr. Dick-Read (one of Margaret Mead's teachers) to ease the pain of contractions during childbirth; involves the father's participation in the birth process.

caesarean section. A surgical operation for delivering a baby by cutting through the mother's abdominal and uterine walls; usually used when there is a perceived risk to the mother and/or child, requiring immediate delivery.

cholesterol. A substance found in animal fats, blood, nerve tissue and bile. High concentrations can lead to atherosclerosis.

DDT. A powerful insecticide currently banned by law due to its damaging effects on environmental and personal health.

eclampsia. A disorder, sometimes occurring in late pregnancy, characterized by convulsions, edema and elevated blood pressure.

ectopic pregnancy. A pregnancy in which the fertilized ovum develops outside the uterus, as in the Fallopian tube.

episiotomy. An incision of the perineum sometimes performed during childbirth to prevent vaginal tearing.

estrogen. Female sex hormones or synthetic compounds that control the menstrual cycle.

HCG. A placental hormone that stimulates the ovaries to produce other hormones that prevent menstruation. Its presence in urine indicates pregnancy.

hematocrit. The proportion of red blood cells to the total volume of blood.

hemoglobin. A red protein in blood which carries oxygen from the lungs to the tissues and carbon dioxide from the tissues to the lungs.

homeostasis. The tendency to maintain internal stability in an organism by coordinated response of organ systems which automatically attempt to compensate for environmental changes.

hypoglycemia. An abnormally low concentration of sugar in the blood.

Kegel exercises. Deliberate contractions of the Kegel muscle which goes from the tail bone to the pubic bone with openings to the bladder, vagina and rectum. Through exercising this muscle, the strength and flexibility of the vaginal area will be increased, reducing the chance of tearing and unnecessary pain during childbirth. Kegel exercises are also used to return the vaginal area to normal size after childbirth.

ketone. An organic chemical compound found in the blood and urine when there is excessive oxidation of fatty acids by the liver.

kwashiorkor. A severe disease of young children caused by a chronic deficiency of protein and calories in the diet resulting in stunted growth, edema and a protuberant belly.

lacto-ovo. Lacto refers to milk, ovo refers to eggs, so a lacto-ovo vegetarian is one who includes eggs and milk/dairy in the diet.

legumes. The seeds of certain plants such as peas and beans which are used as dietary staples throughout most of the world.

leukocyte. Small colorless cells in the blood, lymph and tissues which are important in the body's defenses against infection.

macrobiotic. Refers to a philosophical system originating in Japan which aims to promote a longer, healthier life through balancing the yin and yang elements (the "opposites") in life. It is applied to diet through a very specific regimen that may be vegetarian, but may include seafood as well.

myoglobin. An iron-containing protein in muscle that is similar to hemoglobin, which receives oxygen from red blood cells and transports it to muscle cell mitochondria, where the oxygen is used in cellular respiration to produce energy.

neutropenia. A decrease of white blood cells in the blood, particularly in reaction to various drugs, infections or irradiation.

nitrites. Salts of nitrous acid containing a negative radical.

osteoporosis. A bone disorder characterized by a reduction in bone density accompanied by increasing porosity and brittleness.

oxalates. Salts of oxalic acid containing a negative radical.

PCB. An environmental pollutant found in insulators of electrical equipment.

perineum. The region of the body between the anus and the vagina (or scrotum).

phytates. Salts of phytic acids, phytates are phosphorous compounds found in whole grains, beans and peas. They combine with minerals, especially calcium, iron, and zinc to form insoluble compounds which are then excreted by the body.

placenta abruptio. An abnormal separation of the placenta from the uterus.

placenta previa. An abnormally low placement of the placenta in the uterus, usually on or near the cervix.

pre-eclampsia. The physiological state preceding eclampsia, characterized by hypertension and edema.

progesterone. A steroid hormone active in preparing the uterus for reception and development of the fertilized ovum and the mammary glands for secretion of milk for the newborn baby.

RDA. The Recommended Daily (or Dietary) Allowance, the amount of protein, vitamins and other nutrients suggested for various age groups by the National Food and Nutrition Board.

scurvy. A disease resulting from a deficiency of vitamin C (ascorbic acid) in the diet, characterized by weakness, anemia, puffy gums and bleeding of mucous membranes.

sonogram. A visual pattern produced by sound waves transmitted through the body; used during pregnancy by doctors to determine fetal growth and positioning.

TVP. The acronym for Texturized Vegetable Protein, a protein substance created without any meat products; used in some vegetarian recipes, sold primarily through health food stores.

vegan (vē´gən, vĕj´ən). A vegetarian who eats no animal products (to be pronounced as you like).

Bibliography

Abdulla, M., et al. "Nutrient intake and health status of vegans: Chemical analyses of diets using the duplicate portion sampling technique." *American Journal of Clinical Nutrition* 34:2464–2477; 1981.

Acosta, Phyllis B. "Availability of essential amino acids and nitrogen in vegan diets." *American Journal of Clinical Nutrition* 48:868–74; 1988.

Altman, Lawrence K. "Study finds a vitamin reduces birth defects." *The New York Times* A–14; July 19, 1991.

American Dietetic Association. "Vegetarian diets : Position statement of the American Dietetic Association." *Journal of the American Dietetic Association* 88:3:352–355; 1988.

Anderson, Bonnie M., S. G. Gibson, and J. H. Sabry. "The iron and zinc status of long–term vegetarian women." *American Journal of Clinical Nutrition* 34:1042–1048; 1981.

Apgar, Virginia and Joan Beck. *Is My Baby All Right?* Simon and Schuster, 1972.

Aronson, Virginia. "Can vegetarianism meet your needs?" Chapter 5 in *The Dietetic Technician*. Westport, CT: AVI Publishing Company, 1984.

Ballentine, Rudolph. *Transition to Vegetarianism: An Evolutionary Step.* Pennsylvania: Himalayan International Institute, 1987.

Ballentine, Rudolph. *Diet and Nutrition: A Holistic Approach.* Honesdale, PA: Himalayan International Institute, 1978.

Bargen, Richard. *The Vegetarian's Self–defense Manual.* Wheaton, Illinois: Theosophical Publishing House, 1979.

Bergan, James G. and Phyllis T. Brown. "Nutritional status of 'new' vegetarians." *Journal of the American Dietetic Association* 76:151–155; 1980.

Bloxam, D. L., et al. "Maternal zinc during iron supplementation in pregnancy: a preliminary study." *Clinical Science* 76:59–65; 1988.

Bower, John. *The Healthy House.* Lyle Stuart Publishing, 1989.

Brewer, Gail Sforza and Tom Brewer.*What Every Pregnant Woman Should Know: The Truth About Diets and Drugs in Pregnancy.* Random House, 1977.

Brody, Jane. *Jane Brody's Nutrition Book.* Bantam Books, 1987.

Brody, Jane E. "Eating Well: 3 promising weapons against disease." *The New York Times* C–11; September 25, 1991.

Brown, Judith E. *Nutrition for Your Pregnancy : The University of Minnesota Guide.* Minneapolis: University of Minnesota Press, 1983.

Brown, Judith E. "Improving pregnancy outcomes in the United States: The importance of preventive nutrition services." *Journal of the American Dietetic Association* 89:1:631–633; 1989.

Brown, Judith E. and Mary Story. "'Let Them Eat Cake' or a prescription for improving the outcome of pregnancy: A Response to Nutrition during Pregnancy, Parts I and II" *Nutrition Today* 18–23; November/December 1990.

Burros, Marian. "Dietary Supplements: Let the Buyer Beware." *The New York Times* C–1; October 16, 1991.

Burros, Marian. "A turf war in Washington over food labels." *The New York Times* C–4; October 14, 1992.

Calbom, Cherie and Maureen Keane. *Juicing for Life: A Guide to the Health Benefits of Fresh Fruit and Vegetable Juicing.* New York: Avery Publishing Group, 1992.

Campbell, D.M. and M.D.G. Gillmer, eds. *Nutrition in Pregnancy: Proceedings of the 10th Study Group of the Royal College of Obstetricians and Gynaecologists.* London: Perinatology Press, 1983.

Campion, Mukti Jain. *Baby Challenge: A handbook on pregnancy for women with physical disability.* New York: Routledge, Chapman and Hall, 1990.

Caragay, Alegria. "Cancer–Preventive Foods and Ingredients." *Food Technology* April 1992.

Carlson, E., et al. "A comparative evaluation of vegan, vegetarian and omnivore diets." *Journal of Plant Foods* 6:89–100; 1985.

Carper, Jean. *The Food Pharmacy: Dramatic New Evidence that Food is Your Best Medicine.* Bantam Books, 1988.

Carter, J. P., T. Furman, and H. R. Hutcheson. "Pre–eclampsia and reproductive performance in a community of vegans." *Southern Medical Journal* 80:692–697; 1987.

Chaij–Rhys, S. "A diet pattern for total vegetarians." *Adventist Review* 157:1014–1015; 1980.

Chandra, R.K. "Excessive intake of zinc impairs immune responses." *Journal of the American Medical Association* 252:1443–1446; 1984.

Cherry, Flor F., et al. "Adolescent pregnancy: associations among body weight, zinc nutriture and pregnancy outcome." *American Journal of Clinical Nutrition* 50:945–954; 1989.

Clakins, Beverly M. "Executive summary of the First International Congress on Vegetarian Nutrition." *American Journal of Clinical Nutrition* 48:709–711; 1988.

Clinton, Sally. "What's In Your Cheese?" *Vegetarian Journal* July/August 1991.

"Cocaine–Using Fathers Linked to Birth Defects." *The New York Times* October 15, 1991.

Colbin, Annemarie. *Food and Healing: How what you eat determines your health, your well–being and the quality of your life.* Ballantine Books, 1986.

Committee on Nutrition of the Mother and Preschool Child Food and Nutrition Board. *Alternative Dietary Practices and Nutritional Abuses in Pregnancy.* Washington, D C: National Academy Press, 1982.

Committee on Maternal Nutrition/Food and Nutrition Board/National Research Council. *Maternal Nutrition and the Course of Pregnancy.* Washington, DC: National Academy of Sciences, 1970.

Cook, Lori. *A Shopper's Guide to Cruelty–Free Products.* Bantam, 1991.

Curtis, Glad B. *Your Pregnancy Week–by–Week.* Tucson, AZ: Fisher Books, 1989.

Dadd, Debra Lynn. *Nontoxic Home*. Los Angeles: Jeremy P. Tarcher, 1986.

Dadd, Debra Lynn. *Nontoxic, Natural and Earthwise: How to Protect Yourself and Your Family from Harmful Products*. Los Angeles: Jeremy P. Tarcher, 1990.

Davis, Adelle. *Let's Have Healthy Children*. New American Library, 1972.

"Debating Evening Primrose Oil." *Natural Health* November/December 1992.

DeLyser, Femmy. *Jane Fonda's New Pregnancy Workout and Total Birth Program*. Simon and Schuster, 1991 (1989).

Dwyer, Johanna T. "Health aspects of vegetarian diets." *American Journal of Clinical Nutrition* 48:712–38; 1988.

Eisenberg, Arlene, Heidi Eisenberg Murkoff, and Sandee Eisenberg Hathaway. *What to Eat When You're Expecting*. New York: Workman Publishing, 1986.

Ellis, Frey R. and Montegriffo, V. M. E. "Veganism, clinical findings and investigations." *American Journal of Clinical Nutrition* 23:3:249–255; 1970.

Endres, Jeannette, et al. "Older pregnant women and adolescents: Nutrition data after enrollment in WIC." *Journal of the American Dietetic Association* 87:8:1011–1019; 1987.

Fanelli, M.T. and R. Kuczmarski. "Guidelines for lacto–ovo–vegetarian and vegan diets." in Anderson, J. B., ed., *Nutrition and Vegetarianism: Proceedings of Public Health Nutrition Update*. North Carolina Health Sciences Consortium, 199–206; 1988.

Federal–Provincial Subcommittee on Nutrition, DHEW, Ottawa, Canada. "Canada's national guidelines on prenatal nutrition: Summary Report." *Nutrition Today* 34–35; July/August 1987.

First International Congress on Vegetarian Nutrition. "Proceedings." *American Journal of Clinical Nutrition Supplement* 48:3; 1988.

Fitzpatrick, Elise, et al. *The Pregnancy Nutrition Counter*. Pocket Books, 1992.

"Folic Acid for fighting birth defects?" *Tufts University Diet and Nutrition Letter* 10:9:1–2; 1992.

"Food Guide Pyramid Replaces Basic 4 Circle." *Food Technology* 7:61–64; 1992.

Forsum, Elisabet, A. Sadurskis, and J. Wager. "Resting metabolic rate and body composition of healthy Swedish women during pregnancy." *American Journal of Clinical Nutrition* 47:942–947; 1988.

Freeland–Graves, Jeanne. "Mineral adequacy of vegetarian diets." *American Journal of Clinical Nutrition* 48:859–862; 1988.

Freeland–Graves, Jeanne, et al. "Nutrition knowledge of vegetarians and nonvegetarians." *Journal of Nutritional Education* 14:1:21–26; 1982.

Fried, Peter A. *Pregnancy and Life–Style Habits.* New York: Beaufort Books, 1983.

Frye, Anne. *Understanding Lab Work in the Childbearing Year, 4th ed.: A guide for givers and receivers of health care in childbirth.* New Haven: Labrys Press, 1990.

Fryer, Lee and Dick Simmons. *Whole Foods For You.* New York: Mason & Lipscomb, Publishers, 1974.

Gardner, Joy. *Healing Yourself During Pregnancy.* Freedom, CA: The Crossing Press, 1987.

Goldsmith, Judith. *Childbirth Wisdom From the World's Oldest Societies.* Brookline, MA: East–West Books, 1990.

Goodman, Richard M. *Planning for a Healthy Baby: A Guide to Genetic and Environmental Risks.* New York: Oxford University Press, 1986.

Guthrie, Helen A. "Recommended dietary allowances 1989: Changes, Consensus and Challenges." *Nutrition Today* 43–45; 1990.

Hambridge, K. M., et al. "Acute effects of iron therapy on zinc status during pregnancy." *Obstetrics and Gynecology* 70:593–96; 1987.

Harbarger, Janie Coulter and Neil Harbarger. *Eating for the Eighties: A Complete Guide to Vegetarian Nutrition.* Philadelphia: Saunders Paperbacks, 1981.

Heaney, R. P., C. M. Weaver, and R. R. Recker. "Calcium absorbability from spinach." *American Journal of Clinical Nutrition* 47:707–709; 1988.

Hemminki, Elina and Ulla Rimpela. "A randomized comparison of routine versus selective iron supplementation during pregnancy." *Journal of the American College of Nutrition* 10:1:3–10; 1991.

Herbert, Victor. "Vitamin B–12: plant sources, requirements, and assay." *American Journal of Clinical Nutrition* 48:852–858; 1988.

Hertzler, Ann A., et al. "Development of an iron checklist to guide food intake." *Journal of the American Dietetic Association* 86:6:782–786; 1986.

Hess, Mary Abbott and Anne Elise Hunt. *Pickles & Ice Cream: The Complete Guide to Nutrition During Pregnancy.* McGraw–Hill Book Company, 1982.

Higgins, A.C., et al. "Impact of the Higgins Nutrition Intervention Program on birth weight: a within–mother analysis." *Journal of the American Dietetic Association* 89:8:1097–1103; 1989.

Higginbottom, M.C., L. Sweetman, and W. L. Nyhan. "Syndrome of methylmalonic aciduria, homo cystinuria, megaloblastic anemia and neurological abnormalities in a vitamin B12–deficient breast fed infant of a strict vegetarian." *New England Journal of Medicine* 299:317–323; 1978.

"How do foods affect folate bioavailability?" *Nutrition Reviews* 48:8:326–327; 1990.

Huber, Agnes M., et al. "Folate nutriture in pregnancy." *Journal of the American Dietetic Association* 88:7:791–795; 1988.

Hurd, Frank and Rosalie Hurd. *Ten Talents Cookbook.* Chisholm, TN: The College Press, 1968.

Hurley, Lucille S. *Developmental Nutrition* Prentice–Hall, 1980.

"Inadequate vegan diets at weaning." *Nutrition Reviews* 48:8:323–326; 1990.

Institute of Medicine. *Nutrition During Pregnancy, Part 1: Weight Gain; Part 2: Nutrient Supplements.* Washington, DC: National Academy Press, 1990.

Institute of Medicine. *Nutrition During Pregnancy and Lactation: An Implementation Guide.* Washington, DC: National Academy Press, 1992.

Jackson, Lauren S. and Ken Lee. "The Effect of Dairy Products on Iron Availability." *Critical Review of Food Science and Nutrition* 31(4):259–270; 1992.

Jacobsen, Howard N. "A healthy pregnancy: the struggle to define it." *Nutrition Today* 30–37; 1988.

Jacobson, M. F, L. Y. Lefferts, and A. W. Garland. *Safe Food: Eating Wisely in a Risky World.* Los Angeles: Living Planet Press, 1991.

Johnston, Patricia K. "Counseling the pregnant vegetarian." *American Journal of Clinical Nutrition* 48:901–905; 1988.

Kamen, Betty and Si Kamen. *Total Nutrition During Pregnancy: How To Be Sure You And Your Baby Are Eating The Right Stuff.* New Canaan, CT: Keats Publishing, Inc., 1986.

Kelsay, J. L. and E. S. Prather. "Mineral balances of human subjects consuming spinach in a low–fiber diet and in a diet containing fruits and vegetables." *American Journal of Clinical Nutrition* 38:12–19; 1983.

Kelsay, June L., et al. "Impact of variation in carbohydrate intake on mineral utilization by vegetarians." *American Journal of Clinical Nutrition* 48:875–879; 1988.

King, J. C., T. Stein, and M. Doyle. "Effect of vegetarianism on the zinc status of pregnant women." *American Journal of Clinical Nutrition* June 1981.

Klaper, Michael. *Pregnancy, Children and the Vegan Diet.* Maui, HI: Gentle World, Inc., 1987.

Klein, Diane and Rosalyn T. Badalamenti. *Eating Right for Two: The Complete Nutrition Guide and Cookbook for a Healthy Pregnancy.* Ballantine Books, 1983.

Knight, K. B. and R. E. Keith. "The effect of calcium supplementation on normotensive and hypertensive pregnancy." *American Journal of Clinical Nutrition* 55:891–895; 1992.

Kolata, Gina. "Biologists stumble across new pattern of inheritance." *The New York Times* C-1:7; July 16, 1991.

Kushi, Michio and Aveline Kushi. *Macrobiotic Pregnancy and Care of the Newborn.* New York: Japan Publications, Inc., 1985 (1984).

Lampkin, B. C. and E. F. Saunders. "Nutritional vitamin B12 deficiency in an infant." *Journal of Pediatrics* 75:1053–1055; 1969.

Langley, Gill. *Vegan Nutrition: A Survey of Research.* East Sussex, England: The Vegan Society, 1988.

Leavy, Herbert T., ed. *Vegetarian Times Cookbook by the Editors of Vegetarian Times.* MacMillan Publishing Company, 1984.

Le Tissier, Jackie. *Food Combining for Vegetarians: Eat for Health on the Hay Diet.* London: Thorsons, 1992.

Lettvin, Maggie. *Maggie's Woman's Book: Her Personal Plan for Health and Fitness for Women of Every Age.* Houghton Mifflin, 1980.

Levander, O. A. and Lorraine Cheng, eds. *Micronutrient Interactions: Vitamins, Minerals and Hazardous Elements.* New York Academy of Sciences, 1980.

Lind, T. "Iron Supplementation in Pregnancy." see Campbell, D. M. and M. D. G. Gillmer, *Nutrition in Pregnancy* .

Lloyd, Tom, et al. "Urinary hormonal concentrations and spinal bone densities of premenopausal vegetarian and non–vegetarian women." *American Journal of Clinical Nutrition* 54:1005–1010; 1991.

Lyon, Wendy. *Beautiful Woman's Pregnancy Fitness Book: Nutrition, Diet, Health, Exercise, Beauty, Fashion.* Chicago: Contemporary Books, 1982.

Margen, Sheldon, et al. *Wellness Encyclopedia of Food and Nutrition.* Random House, 1992.

McCartney, Marion and Antonia van der Meer. *The Midwife's Pregnancy and Childbirth Book: Having Your Baby Your Way.* Harper and Row, 1991.

McMahon, Judi, with exercises by Zia Odell. *A Year of Beauty and Exercise for the Pregnant Woman: A Month–by–Month Guide to Looking and Feeling Your Joyful Best.* Lippincott and Crowell, Publishers, 1980.

Michaud, Ellen, et al. *Listen to your Body: A Head–to–Toe Guide to More than 400 Symptoms, Their Causes and Best Treatments* Emmaus, PA: Rodale Press, 1988.

Miller, Benjamin F. *The Complete Medical Guide.* Simon & Schuster, 1978.

Mitchell, Mary C. and Edith Lerner. "Weight gain and pregnancy outcome in underweight and normal weight women." *Journal of the American Dietetic Association* 89:5:634–641; 1989.

Mitra, Ananda. *Food for Thought: The Vegetarian Philosophy.* Willow Springs, MO: Nucleus Publications, 1991.

Moghissi, K. and T. Evans, eds. "Factors in Intrauterine Impoverishment." in *Nutritional Impacts on Women.* Harper and Row, 1977.

Monsen, Elaine R. "Iron nutrition and absorption: Dietary factors which impact iron bioavailability." *Journal of the American Dietetic Association* 88:7:786–790; 1988.

Munoz, Leda, et al. "Coffee consumption as a factor in iron deficiency anemia among pregnant women and their infants in Costa Rica." *American Journal of Clinical Nutrition* 48:645–651; 1988.

Mutch, Patricia B. "Food guides for the vegetarian." *American Journal of Clinical Nutrition* 48:913–919; 1988.

Nathanielsz, Peter W. *Life Before Birth.* Ithaca, NY: Promethean Press, 1992.

Nathanielsz, Peter W. *A Time to Be Born.* Ithaca, NY: Promethean Press, 1992.

National Institute of Nutrition (Canada). "Risks and benefits of vegetarian diets." *Nutrition Today* 27–29 March/April 1990.

National Research Council. *Recommended Dietary Allowances, 10th Edition* Washington, DC: National Academy Press, 1989.

Nielsen, Suzanne S. "Digestibility of Legume Proteins." *Food Technology* 9:112–118; 1991.

Nightingale, Elena O. and Melissa Goodman. *Before Birth: Prenatal Testing for Genetic Disease.* Cambridge, MA: Harvard University Press, 1990.

Nilsson, Lennart. *A Child is Born.* Delacorte Press, 1990.

Norwood, Christopher. *At Highest Risk: Protecting Children from Environmental Injury.* Penguin Books, 1980.

Nutrition Search, Inc. *Nutrition Almanac.* McGraw–Hill Book Company, 1992.

Parham, Ellen S., et al. "The association of pregnancy weight gain with the mother's postpartum weight." *Journal of the American Dietetic Association* 90:4:550–554; 1990.

Park, Youngmee K., et al. "Characteristics of vitamin and mineral supplement products in the U.S." *American Journal of Clinical Nutrition* 54:750–759; 1991.

Parvati, Jeannine. *Hygieia: A Woman's Herbal.* Berkeley, CA: self–published, 1978.

Peacok, Munro. "Calcium absorption efficiency and calcium requirements for children and adults." *American Journal of Clinical Nutrition* 54:2615–2655; 1991.

Phillips, R. D. and K. H. McWatters. "Contribution of Cowpeas to Nutrition and Health." *Food Technology* September 1991.

"Pre-eclampsia Prevention." *Prevention* 9:29–30; 1992.

Reece, Janet, P. R. Donovan, and A. Y. Pellett. "Iron supplementation in pregnancy: Testing a clinic protocol." *Journal of the American Dietetic Association* 87:12:1682–1683; 1987.

Repke, John T. and J. Villar. "Pregnancy–induced hypertension and low birth weight: the role of calcium." *American Journal of Clinical Nutrition* 54:2375–2415; 1991.

Reynolds, Robert D. "Bioavailability of vitamin B–6 from plant foods." *American Journal of Clinical Nutrition* 48:863–867; 1988.

Ridgway, Roy. *Caring for Your Unborn Child: How to give your baby the best. possible start in life.* London: Thorsons, 1990.

Robertson, Laurel, C. Flinders, and B. Godfrey. *Laurel's Kitchen: A Handbook for Vegetarian Cookery and Nutrition, 2nd ed.* Berkeley, California: Ten Speed Press, 1986.

Rosso, Pedro. *Nutrition and Metabolism in Pregnancy: Mother and Fetus.* New York: Oxford University Press, 1990.

Savage, G. P. "Nutritional value of sprouted mung beans." *Nutrition Today* 21–24; May/June 1990.

Scher, Jonathan and Carol Dix. *Will My Baby Be Normal? How to Make Sure: Everything You Need to Know About Pregnancy.* Dial Press, 1983.

Schneck, Mary E., et al. "Low–income pregnant adolescents and their infants: Dietary findings and health outcomes." *Journal of the American Dietetic Association* 90:4:555–558; 1990.

Schoemaker, Joyce and Charity Vitale. *Healthy Homes, Healthy Kids.* Washington, D. C.: Island Press, 1991.

Scholl, Theresa, et al. "Anemia vs. Iron Deficiency: Increased risk of preterm delivery in a prospective study." *American Journal of Clinical Nutrition* 55:985–988; 1992.

Schwartz, Leni. *World of the Unborn: Nurturing your child before birth.* New York: Richard Marek Publishers, 1980.

Seamens, Dan. "Moosewood Revisited." *Natural Health* November/December 1992.

Seamens, Dan. "Eating for Optimum Health: Is there a place for animal food in the healthy diet?" *Natural Health* November/December 1992.

Sha, Janet L. *Mothers of Thyme: Customs and Rituals of Infertility and Miscarriage.* Ann Arbor, MI: Lida Rose Press, 1990.

Shaffer, Willa. *Midwifery and Herbs.* Provo, UT: Woodland Books, 1986.

Shapiro, Eben. "The Long, Hard Quest for Foods that Fool the Palate." *The New York Times* September 29, 1991.

Shapiro, Eben. "Food Industry Views the Thrifty Bean with New Admiration." *The New York Times* C–3: September 2, 1991.

Sharop, F., R. B. Fraser, and R. D. B. Milner, eds. *Fetal Growth.* London: Springer–Verlag, 1989.

Sheldon, W. L., et al. "The effects of oral iron supplementation on zinc and magnesium levels during pregnancy." *British Journal of Obstetrics and Gynaecology* 92:892–898; 1985.

Shurtleff, William and Akiko Aoyagi. *The Book of Tofu.* Ballantine Books, 1988.

Shurtleff, William and Akiko Aoyagi. *The Book of Miso*. Ballantine Books, 1988 (1976).

Small, Meredith F. "Sperm Wars." *Discover* 48–53; July 19, 1991.

Smotherman, William P., and Scott R. Robinson, eds. *Behavior of the Fetus*. Caldwell, NJ: Telford Press, 1988.

Sonberg, Lynn. *The A to Z Guide to Toxic Foods and How to Avoid Them*. Pocket Books, 1992.

Specker, Bonny L., et al. "Increased urinary methylmalonic acid excretion in breast–fed infants of vegetarian mothers and identification on an acceptable dietary source of vitamin B–12." *American Journal of Clinical Nutrition* 47:89–92; 1988.

Spiller, Gene A. "Beyond Dietary Fiber." *American Journal of Clinical Nutrition* 54:615–617; 1991.

Srikumar, T. S., et al. "Trace element status in healthy subjects switching from a mixed to a lactovegetarian diet for 12 months." *American Journal of Clinical Nutrition* 55:885–90; 1992.

Stautberg, Susan Schiffer. *Pregnancy Nine to Five: The Career Woman's Guide to Pregnancy and Motherhood*. Simon and Schuster, 1985.

Stepaniak, Joanne and Kathy Hecker. *Ecological Cooking: Recipes to Save the Planet*. Ann Arbor: Edwards Brothers Inc., 1991.

Stowers, Sharon L. "Development of a culturally appropriate food guide for pregnant Caribbean immigrants in the U.S." *Journal of the American Dietetic Association* 3:331–336; 1992.

Subcommittee on Nutritional Status and Weight Gain During Pregnancy and the Subcommittee on Dietary Intake and Nutrient Supplements During Pregnancy. "Nutrition during pregnancy: Executive Summary." *Nutrition Today* 13–22; July/August 1990.

Suitor, C. W., et al. "Characteristics of diet among a culturally diverse group of low–income pregnant women." *Journal of the American Dietetic Association* 90:4:543–549; 1990.

Sussman, John and B. Blake Levitt. *Before You Conceive: The Complete Prepregnancy Guide*. Bantam Books, 1989.

Swanson, B. G. and J. Cash. "Symposium: Processing, Food Value and Health Benefits." *Food Technology* 9:96–130; 1991.

Task Force on Nutrition Assessment of Maternal Nutrition. American Dietetic Association 1978.

Thomson, Bill. "Essential Fatty Acids in Fish: the Heart Protectors." *Natural Health* November/December 1992.

Vobecky, Jitka S. "Nutritional aspects of preconceptual period as related to pregnancy and early infancy." *Progress in Food and Nutrition Science* 10:205–236; 1986.

Wasserman, Debra. *Simply Vegan: Quick Vegetarian Meals.* Baltimore: Vegetarian Resource Group, 1991.

Weaver, C. M., et al. "Human calcium absorption from whole–wheat products." *Journal of Nutrition* 121:1769–1775; 1991.

Weed, Susun S. *Wise Woman Herbal for the Childbearing Year.* New York: Ash Tree Publishing, 1986.

Whelan, Elizabeth M. *Pregnancy Experience: A Psychological Guide for Expectant Parents* W. W. Norton & Company, 1978.

Wilcox, A. J. and C. R. Weinberg. "Tea and Fertility." *Lancet* 337:1159–1160; 1991.

Willensky, Diana. "Easing Severe Morning Sickness." *American Health* 9:86; 1992.

Williams, Phyllis. *Nourishing Your Unborn Child: Nutrition and Natural Foods in Pregnancy.* Avon Books, 1982 (1974).

Windham, C. T., A. A. Helm, and W. W. Bonita. "Integrity of small data bases in computer analysis of dietary data." *Food Science and Nutrition* 29:3:149–166; 1990.

Winter, Ruth. *Consumer's Dictionary of Household, Yard and Office Chemicals.* Crown Publishing, 1992.

Worth, Cecilia. *Health and Beauty During Pregnancy.* McGraw–Hill Book Company, 1984.

Worthington–Roberts, Bonnie S. "Nutrition and maternal health." *Nutrition Today* 6–19; November/December 1984.

Worthington–Roberts, Bonnie S. and Sue Rodwell Williams. *Nutrition in Pregnancy and Lactation, 4th Edition.* St. Louis: C. V. Mosby Company, 1989.

Worthington–Roberts, Bonnie S., ed. *Contemporary Developments in Nutrition.* St. Louis: C. V. Mosby Company, 1981.

Wrench, G. T. *The Wheel of Health.* London: C. W. Daniel Company, Ltd., 1938.

Yasodhara, P., L. A. Ramaraju, and L. Raman. "Trace minerals in pregnancy: Copper and Zinc." *Nutrition Research* 11:15–21; 1991.

Zemel, Michael B. "Calcium utilization: effect of varying level and source of dietary protein." *American Journal of Clinical Nutrition* 48:880–883; 1988.

Index

About the Author

Sharon K. Yntema was born in Detroit, Michigan in 1951 and grew up on St. Croix in the U.S. Virgin Islands where her mother first introduced her to a vegetarian diet. She received a B.A. in Psychology from Earlham College and an M.A. in Early Childhood Special Education from George Washington University. Before her son was born in 1978, she worked as a child development specialist at the Day Care and Child Development Council in Ithaca, New York. She still lives in Ithaca where she works as the buyer/bookkeeper for a large independent bookstore. Her vegetarian son continues to be very healthy, smart and tall, having passed his mother's 5'8" stature by age 14.